BLuSh

BLUSH

A MEMOIR

HOW I BARELY SURVIVED 17

Danielle Ripley-Burgess

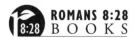

ROMANS 8:28 BOOKS

Cover concept and design by Will Bryan Design.

Published by Romans 8:28 Books, an imprint of Redemption Press, PO Box 427, Enumclaw, WA 98022.

Toll-Free (844) 2REDEEM (273-3336)

Redemption Press is honored to present this title in partnership with the author. The views expressed or implied in this work are those of the author. Redemption Press provides our imprint seal representing design excellence, creative content, and high-quality production.

Unless otherwise noted, Scripture quotations are taken from the Holy Bible, New International Version®, NIV® Copyright ©1973, 1978, 1984, 2011 by Biblica, Inc.® Used by permission. All rights reserved worldwide.

Scripture quotations marked NLT are taken from the Holy Bible, New Living Translation, copyright © 1996, 2004, 2015 by Tyndale House Foundation. Used by permission of Tyndale House Publishers Inc., Carol Stream, Illinois 60188. All rights reserved.

ISBN: 978-1-64645-126-5 (Paperback)
978-1-64645-127-2 (ePub)
978-1-64645-131-9 (Mobi)

Library of Congress Catalog Card Number: 2020904283

For Mae
Never be afraid to use your voice and speak your truth.

AUTHOR'S NOTE

BEYOND DECADES OF JOURNAL ENTRIES, I have relied on my family's memory to describe several scenes interspersed over two decades. Also, readers may notice the chapters aren't totally chronological—an editing decision for narrative flow. And as this is a survivorship memoir, certain medical procedures I describe may be slightly outdated. Finally, I touch on several topics related to puberty, so parents, I encourage you to have "the talk" with your daughters or sons before they read this, unless you're hoping to avoid the conversation, in which case this book will unabashedly start to explain it.

CONTENTS

PROLOGUE

Aisle 7

No way I was backing down. With my Converse sneakers glued to the sticky retail floor, I glared back into my mom's eyes—my protest in the middle of the Walmart toilet paper aisle was *on*. I clamped my outstretched arms over the basket of our shopping cart.

"No. Absolutely not!"

Like two gladiators in a packed coliseum, we fixed our squinty-eyed gazes and cocked our heads. A battle of wills broke out as we both made ourselves perfectly clear: *Today, I'm in control.*

The fluorescent lightbulbs buzzed above, making everything in the store shiny. High-stacked boxes of white plastic silverware and rows of zippered sandwich bags watched over us as my arms formed a canopy over our cart. The makeshift barricade kept the toilet paper *out* and the remnants of my pride *in*.

Mom stood silent at first. I assumed she saw me as a typical bratty preteen who couldn't rightly be reasoned with. I could tell she was angry, but she didn't yell. Like a hula dancer about to begin her routine, she shifted her weight to one hip, then stopped. Her hands slid up and rested on her hips.

This is war, I assumed she was thinking, although I didn't care to really know or understand.

Game on was my unspoken reply.

I stood my ground, glaring back into her hazel-green eyes—the exact color I saw when I looked at my own in the mirror. For most of my twelve years, I'd been told we looked *sooo* much alike. With dark, long hair and fair, freckled skin, we drew a lot of comments from people we did and didn't know. Our uncanny resemblance had even made us semifinalists in a local newspaper look-alike contest when I was in second grade. We spent the weeks leading up to the photo shoot choosing our matching outfits. We landed on black-and-white striped shirts with a three-scrunchie ponytail hairdo.

"You could be sisters!" the photographer kept saying.

I looked at the camera and smiled politely. At eight years old, I didn't mind looking like Mom. I liked being the same. I belonged with Mom, and that made me feel good. But four short years later, things changed. We were different now, and I didn't want to be like her anymore. I had my own opinions about life. About beauty. About God. And about toilet paper in our shopping cart!

Other shoppers wearing high school team sweat-shirts or logos of Kansas City sports teams gave us polite, uncomfortable smiles and gently steered their carts around us. They were sporting traditional attire seen around the suburbs full of middle-class families like ours, flush with manicured lawns and strip malls. Not quite the big city, yet not rural farm acreage, these Missouri suburbs were the epitome of safe. Mostly conservative. And family friendly. This had been the backdrop of my entire life.

Announcements calling workers to the busy checkouts had turned into dull background noises, as did the kiddo cries a few aisles over signaling they didn't get to put sugar-laden cereals in their shopping carts.

Just wait, kids, I thought. *It's going to get much worse.*

My arms shook a little as my muscles tired, but I didn't move. Couldn't back down now. I assumed the surging hormones responsible for my bumpy chest, vining leg hair, and curving hips were to blame for the standoff—at least from my side of the aisle. A new set of feelings had begun to emerge, and I felt gutsier, more willing to test my limits. For once, I was willing to break the rules. I was the firstborn child; this was not like me. I had never protested my mom's shopping list before. I was known to behave like a perfect angel. In fact, she'd nicknamed me Angel Face because I was so different from my rowdy brother, Andy, not even thirteen months younger. But after only a few weeks of sixth grade, the well of emotions I'd tried to hold back erupted like lava. I thought, felt, and acted differently—already I wasn't sure who was the real me. I couldn't help it either—it just started happening.

It would take many years before I'd realize this was normal behavior for a twelve-year-old girl. In becoming young women, it's normal to break away from our moms and find our own definitions of beauty and of being a lady. But I didn't know that then. All I knew was womanhood didn't mix with the bathroom. The way I saw it, *any*thing involving the bathroom was gross. Bathrooms were for immature boys, men, and dads who laughed at farts, butts, and whoopee cushions. They were for dudes who yanked up their belts and strolled to the toilet after a big Thanksgiving meal during halftime to get a laugh about what came next. Gross. I couldn't imagine my aunts and grandmas receiving the same response had they acted the same way. I knew they used the restroom. Everybody did. But the ladies never drew attention to it. Girls using the restroom were quiet and sly.

"Don't you think *every*one uses toilet paper?"

The silence broke with Mom's whisper, but I shook my head no. I refused to show her any agreement. My arms, still covering our shopping cart, now thrummed with pain. They felt as heavy as the five-pound sacks of potatoes we'd passed near the produce aisle. Light rock music filled the air, but I didn't pay it any attention. I didn't notice anything except the panic-filled thoughts racing through my mind. "What if someone sees me here, and we have toilet paper in our cart? I would die!"

After all, this was the truth of my standoff—a plea for dignity and honor. A longing to fit in when, truth be told, I felt so alone. But I couldn't let any of that leave my lips, mostly because I didn't realize that all those feelings lay behind my behavior. Clearly Mom didn't get it, or she would have given up. As each second passed and the standoff grew longer, so did the distance between us. I longed for her to remember what growing up felt like and send me an empathetic look, or even a smile. But it never came—the war raged on.

The funny thing: I'd waged a war out of fear someone would see us buying toilet paper, yet I was willing to cause a scene on aisle 7. I wasn't acting logically, or I would have let my trembling arms down and moved out of the way far sooner. Yet I was on a mission, and stubbornness wasn't allowing me, or her, to back down. What she couldn't see was my confusion and discomfort that accompanied the onset of my changes. Who was she to me? Who was I to her? I really didn't know anymore.

The frost on the frozen foods transformed into water droplets. New background noise of rattling carts and laughs from other shoppers broke through. Though the standoff had been underway for only a minute or two, it felt like hours. Mom continued to stand across the cart, gladiator to gladiator, determined to prevail. She didn't want to make a second trip just to buy toilet paper, and deep down I didn't blame her. But she could never know—she could not win.

Exhausted and frustrated, I began to show fatigue. With sighs and more hula-hip shifts, Mom did the same. But eventually, her will showed itself to be stronger than mine. The familiar cocked head and pursed lips told me the match was over. I feared what would come next if I didn't move out of her way. I didn't like it when she got unhappy. With a sigh of defeat and a nasty look for good measure, I moved my arms just in time for the double-ply rolls to land atop the soggy pot pies.

"But I am *not* carrying it to the car," I insisted as I

crossed my arms and tucked my fists into my armpit-holsters. I had no other place for my anger to go. I clenched my jaw, bottling my frustration.

She will never understand me, I told myself. *No use to even try.* With my head hung low and cheeks blushing, I followed my mom to the checkout lane. My heart raced. My eyes scanned left to right not for canned goods or lunchbox snacks, but for lurking friends from school whom I feared would see me. And our cart.

This is the worst day of my life, I thought as we made our way to the car to load up the groceries. Keeping my promise, I refused to touch the twelve rolls of shrink-wrapped toilet paper. Luckily, no one had seen me at the store, but I still stewed the whole way home, angry and hurt. Defeated.

"I'm never going to the store again . . . at least if TP is on the list," I said under my breath to calm my thoughts. And I didn't budge on this—keeping my promise for years while avoiding buying toilet paper at every turn. Mom obliged by shopping solo when it was on her list. Getting out of those trips should have been one of my greatest adolescent victories, as I'd actually stood my ground. I'd stood up for what *I* wanted, what I thought I needed. I'd stepped into the extraordinary, even if for a moment, and found my voice. While I'd lost the battle in Walmart that day, as the weeks played out it felt as if I'd won the war. Unfortunately, the victory didn't last long. In a few years, I'd come to realize that TP in a shopping cart was the *least* of my worries.

PART 1

1

The Video

I'VE CALLED KANSAS CITY "HOME" all my life. While I don't remember the first three years, I'm told they were spent in the Green House, a ranch-style home our family owned in the eighties. We lived in the heart of the city before selling the house and moving to the suburban south.

Thanks to thriving blue-ribbon schools, a revitalized downtown, and well-kept parks, people have raved over our suburban town for as long as I can remember. For starters, a downtown diner served cinnamon rolls as appetizers. Early in elementary school, I learned that a Confederate robber named Cole Younger, who ran with the infamous Jesse James after the Civil War, was also from my hometown. At the time, he was our city's biggest claim to fame, even if he was an outlaw. In an odd way, he gave me hope. People who grew up in suburbs in the middle of the USA had, well, a shot at making history books. Maybe that was why my mom agreed one fall afternoon to accompany me to the cemetery that sits in the middle of town and snap a photo of me behind Cole Younger's crumbling concrete grave. I cherished the photo for years. It was a reminder that extraordinary people could come from ordinary places. People like me.

"We moved out here for the schools," my dad consistently said when welcoming guests into our modest three-bedroom yellow house and explaining what had led us to the suburbs. It was part of a story I cherished no matter how many times he (or my mom) told it.

"We met at college in northeast Missouri during business school," one of my parents would often say. And then the details trailed of how they dated, left behind their small Missouri towns, got married, and then moved to Kansas City for jobs.

I loved hearing the origins of my family's story of how and why we landed in Kansas City—it almost always led to the cold December night I made my grand entrance.

"There was a blizzard, it was almost Christmas, and I was studying for my insurance test." Dad would grin as he told about the night I was born.

"We were so glad to have you because we struggled to get pregnant because of endometriosis," Mom often chimed in (cueing my gagging sound and puke face).

Dad would continue the story. "When I got home from the hospital that night, I walked in the front door and spilled the nuggets I'd ordered from the drive-through all over the floor. I was so tired, I just sat there and ate them."

Dad would laugh at himself, which triggered more of Mom's memories.

"Your eyes were wide open, and you looked around the hospital room once they got you swaddled. The nurses had never seen a baby so alert after being born!"

I'd smile proudly; it felt awesome to be unique from the start. Pleasing and "pleasantly surprising" adults became a reputation I never let down. According to notes Mom scribbled in my leather-bound photo album, I hit my developmental milestones on time and delighted all who met me. There were pictures of me on a blanket, pictures of me playing with my favorite toys, and pictures of me sleeping soundly in my wooden crib. Without a peep, I let friends, family, and neighbors all snuggle and hold me.

Mom always loved taking pictures, and they chronicled the details of our lives. From mundane moments of me playing with a laundry basket in our Green House to the adventures we had at the zoo and the Kansas City Plaza, the photos showed me getting bigger and bigger—something that was also happening to Mom's belly. In the midst of my announced accomplishments like "Danielle potty trained herself at thirteen months old!" another little human Ripley appeared.

"Danielle is a great big sister to her baby brother, Andy!" read the caption under the photo of a one-year-old me holding an eight-pound baby brother.

In memories that exist only through photos and stories, just weeks after I turned one, I had a constant companion. He looked a lot like me and my parents, with his jet-black hair and fair skin. At first Andy and I were two peas in a pod. Matching outfits, pool playtime, and riding on our plastic horse, Clip Clop, we were practically always together. Andy was my close playmate and friend. But over time, something changed. I realized he was a gross and annoying *boy*. As we got older, he became a challenger and opponent. It didn't matter if it was across plastic Battleship boards or a deck of cards and a game of war, the two peas in a pod evolved and became more like cats and dogs. As we grew into our individual personalities, we couldn't have been more different.

Andy was boisterous and rowdy; I was quiet and shy. I followed the rules; he liked to test them. Andy loved Chiefs football and outside stuff like hunting and camping. I preferred staying inside, making art, and going to museums and libraries. Not only were our hobbies and personalities different, our health adventures were quite different too. I rarely got sick, with the exception of the chicken pox, and visited the hospital only one time. I had hit my head on the edge of our porcelain bathtub and needed stitches smack in my right eyebrow.

"I thought you were going to go into shock!" my mom later told me as she watched me shake and turn white in the ER. The thought of needles, bleeding, and a doctor sewing me up nearly had me undone. It was all very new for me, but not for them—because of Andy. The hospital was pretty much his scene.

As a baby, he was born with clubfoot, which required multiple major surgeries before he turned six. This had gotten us all used to things like wheelchair ramps, casts, stitches, scars, and bloody bandages. But outside of his foot surgeries, Andy was also accident prone.

"Mom, I sliced my finger on the neighbor's mailbox as I rode by it on my bike," he said as he ran into the house one summer afternoon, which led to a row of black stitches and hours in the emergency room.

"Hurry. Get in the car. Your brother smashed his finger moving a big rock at Boy Scout camp" came the reason for another hospital trip several summers later.

One time, an ER visit of his was actually my fault.

"Andy jumped out of the tree and can't move his arm!" I said while rushing into my great-grandparents' living room. We'd been visiting my mom's grandparents and got permission to play outside after we couldn't take any more sitting still in the dark living room, which smelled like pipe tobacco and old people. We found a perfect climbing tree in the front yard and quickly scaled its branches. After a while, I wanted to go inside for a Little Debbie Star Crunch, something they'd promised us if we were good. So I hopped out of the tree. I looked up into the branches, trying to get Andy to follow. He hesitated, but I insisted.

"Come on, jump! Are you *chick*en? Come on, chicken, jump!"

I wasn't usually so mean, but I really wanted the treat. Never would he have been taunted had I known that once he jumped and hit ground, he'd break his arm, need a cast, and visit yet another set of doctors.

It was odd that Andy and I were so different, since we were practically always together. Being only one grade apart, we attended the same schools and the same Sunday school classes, and since we both had winter birthdays, we even shared some of our parties.

"Happy birthday, Dear Danielle . . . and Andy . . . happy birthday to you!"

Mom had rented a party table at the skating rink to help our birthdays feel special. We each got to invite a handful of friends, and we filled the mustard-colored benches with half boys and half girls. The spinning disco ball, plus pop music bouncing off the painted cinderblock walls, distracted me from the reality that it wasn't just *my* party. My friends didn't seem to mind as much as I did, and the further distraction of doing the limbo on roller skates—*whoa*—eventually helped me get over it.

Although I often would have loved a party of my own, or a life without my younger brother around all the time, I eventually began to accept him. Because we were close to the same age, we learned how to entertain ourselves and coexist. We'd spend hours playing Nintendo or tossing the football across the backyard with our neighbor, Dave. I eventually started to like my little bro, although I would have never said that out loud. When we sat side by side trying to rescue a pink princess in Mario Brothers or race around the bases at the baseball diamond, I'd recognize how much we needed each other and how fun he was. While I wanted always to be older and wiser, when we'd play together, I'd recognize how we were pretty much the same. Unfortunately, this all came crashing down when puberty entered our lives.

I assumed it was going to be an ordinary fall school night—one where I'd head outside shortly after getting off the bus and grab a handful of chocolate chip cookies from our cookie jar for an after-school snack. I didn't think much about the changing seasons, but I did love the crisp air of fall. Because the weather hadn't yet turned cold, the neighborhood kids and I had big plans after school. Our yellow house was in a newly built subdivision and conveniently backed up to one of the prestigious city parks. Backyards of all our neighbors bordered the park, which incubated us as we played. A mini-paradise where we could all run freely. Besides evergreens and climbing trees, the park had a shelter house with picnic tables, a full-size basketball court, a dirt-filled baseball diamond, and our favorite, a wooden swing set surrounded by sand. Because the park was practically hidden in our neighborhood, few people knew about it, and we almost always had it to ourselves.

Each afternoon, all of us kids from the neighborhood would get off our bus and meet in the park after school to play before it got dark outside. One night before I ran out to meet my friends, Mom stopped me and said I needed to come home early. "Tonight you and I are going to a program at your old school. We got a letter about it. It's just for us girls."

She pointed to a single-page typed letter sitting on the kitchen counter inviting us to a girls-only evening. This was new. I wanted to play in the park, but I also liked the idea of a night for just Mom and me. I craved her attention and approval; time to be alone, as just us girls, sounded really fun.

"All the fourth-grade girls and their moms are invited."

Strange, I thought. But fourth grade was starting to

bring new things, and this must be one of them. Thanks to my teacher, I'd been encouraged to write more mini-books and plays, which she then let me share with our class. Mom and Dad also trusted me with more responsibility. They gave me an old stereo to set up in my room, and unbeknownst to them, I wasn't listening to Christian cassette tapes but Top 40 radio and pop songs. Although I still wanted to play outside with the neighborhood kids each afternoon, fourth grade was also bringing new feelings. Sometimes people called me a "tween." I assumed that was right—as long as it meant I wasn't a little kid anymore, yet not yet a full-blown teen.

"Sounds fun . . . I'll be back soon!" Making sure Mom knew I wanted to attend our program, I squeezed at least a little bit of playing time.

An hour or so later, Mom's loud voice echoed off the neighbors' houses and every tree trunk. "Danielllllllleeeeee! Annnnddddyyyyy!"

It was our signal to run home. We couldn't miss it (nor could anyone else within a half mile). She was the loudest mom on the block—she'd later call it her "teacher voice." Dinner was ready for us on the stove once we got inside and washed our hands, a big pot of spaghetti and meat sauce. I loaded up my plate; it was one of my favorite meals Mom made. We usually ate around the table, but since Mom and I had plans, we ate in shifts. After quickly clearing my plate, I loaded it into the dishwasher. (I was careful to do all the chores Mom asked so I could remain her Angel Face.)

Anticipation turned into excitement as girls-only night drew closer. In the car on the way to the event, I wondered what it could be.

Music? Clothes to try on? Nail polish or makeovers?

I hadn't attended anything like this before except Girl Scout functions, which I didn't love so much. I wasn't really into camping, hiking, or using the restroom in port-a-potties. I hoped *this* would be fun!

Turned out a school not too far from our house—in fact, the one I used to attend—was hosting the event. As we pulled into the parking lot, I started to reminisce. Mrs. High's kind voice and pretty handwriting in kindergarten. Losing my teeth in Mrs. G's first grade. Making ice cream in coffee cans we rolled down the playground. Now, in a "historic" school setting, I was ready to make even more memories! How cool.

After parking and getting inside, we saw signs telling us we needed to be in the library. Remembering the way, I felt pride as Mom followed me, and I immediately recognized the short tables pushed to the sides of the room once we walked in. Dozens of chairs were lined up for some type of mini-assembly. It certainly wasn't arranged for the spa night I had in my mind.

Looking around, I realized not much had changed. The wall posters reminding me to read books and stay off drugs were the same. The school's computer lab still sat in the corner, set apart with glass windows and a wooden door.

"This is a floppy disk. See how it flops around?"

I remembered our computer lab teacher's lesson on file storage well. He'd asked our class to huddle around him so we could hear the jiggling noise. I hadn't seen a holey floppy disk actually *flop* since that day. Though it hadn't been that long ago, a lot about computers had already changed. The floppy disks like the one my teacher showed us had been replaced by small, rigid plastic disks (which, weirdly enough, were still called floppy disks). Adults often talked about something called the "internet" being on its way.

Noise in the library got louder, and I looked for other friends or even moms I knew, but nobody stood out. I recognized a few girls who played in my softball league, but none from my team. I started to get a funny feeling in my stomach.

Why exactly are we here?

"Welcome, and thank you for coming!"

A cheery woman with hot-rollered brown hair walked to the front of the room and stood in front of the TV cart. She was wearing a lot of makeup, a fancy dress, and tall high heels. Motioning for us to take a seat, she said the program would soon begin. Mom and I followed directions. As the room hushed, the lady returned and explained the purpose of our invitation: we were going to watch a movie about growing up. The funny feeling wasn't so funny anymore. *This* was the exciting girls night? Boring.

"Can someone get the lights?"

The video began.

At the sound of a tape winding through the VCR, the TV screen lit up with a scene featuring teenage girls sitting on their bikes, talking. My eyes perked up. At ten years old, I liked riding bikes. Even more, I liked watching older teenage girls. I listened in.

"My mom said my chest is growing, and I need a bra . . ."

"My mom said I'm going through something called puberty."

Puberty? This wasn't bike talk. Or was it? Shuffling uncomfortably in my chair, I looked away. My attention turned to reading titles on book spines, but the video's offscreen narrator got me to once again look up. "These are fallopian tubes. Each month an egg is released . . ."

On the screen, illustrations of girls' organs had lines and labels pointing to each part. Animations explained that as girls grow up, they release eggs each month and go through a process called "menstruation." I vaguely knew what this meant—period stuff. Mom had very briefly mentioned it, but this video was *way* more in depth. Wanting to barf, I looked around the room to see if any of the other girls looked as awkward as I felt, but it was so dark, I couldn't tell. The video played on.

Puberty didn't just happen to the girls on TV; it was going to happen to me! Ohhhhh no.

More animations that showed little white eggs moving through things that looked like alien tentacles officially freaked me out. It was especially scary to learn what happened to "wash out" the unfertilized egg every month. Blood. I don't know if it was a graphic or the way the narrator said it, but in one split second, everything clicked. I realized why the school was hosting the video for Mom and me.

Puberty didn't just happen to the girls on TV; it was going to happen to me! Ohhhhh no.

I bit my tongue to stay quiet. On the inside, I panicked. *Why are the teenage girls on their bikes so happy? This is* horr*ible!*

I needed a distraction, so I let my eyes wander again to the bookshelves. More memories of sitting with my kindergarten class came to mind. I remembered a favorite book I checked out often, one about a girl's routine for cleaning her room. The book was patterned, and everything had a place. In the story, nothing went wrong. Everything ended up happy. If only I could have transported into her story, or even back to kindergarten days. But that wasn't an option, and neither was going through puberty. Scared and disgusted, I slouched into my seat.

"Okay, moms and daughters . . ."

The video finally ended, which meant cheery high-heel lady was back. The lights flipped on, but none of us girls dared to look around the room or make eye contact. It was so awkward. Cheery lady's voice was an octave higher than it had been before the video played. She clearly liked talking about puberty, but I was done. Unceremoniously, the evening finally ended.

"Questions?" Mom's voice broke the near silence, the calming sound of our tires humming along the highway. Our drive home was quick, our conversation about the evening even quicker. I was glad Mom couldn't see the sour expression on my face, although my attitude likely told her how I felt.

"No, I'm good," I lied.

I did have questions, a lot of them. But I didn't know how or what to ask. Disappointed that the evening had gone nothing like what I'd expected, and scared about puberty, I didn't want to talk. Why didn't I get a say in what my body did? Why did it have to be so gross? I felt a lot of things, but I didn't want to share.

Looking down, I fumbled with the zipper on a pink goodie bag in my hands. Cheery lady had insisted we take one on our way out. It was full of things I didn't consider good (or spa-like), things called tampons and pads. Holding them in my hands made everything in the video feel so final. So real. I wanted to toss it in the trash, but I didn't want to be rude.

By the time we got home, it was late and dark. Fortunately, my brother was already in his bedroom. I'd been nervous to see him after watching the video. Actually, I didn't want to be around any boys. Did they know what girls' bodies did? Did it freak them out as much as it did me? I couldn't shake the fear and shame that came each time I thought about my body and what the video said it would one day do.

Dad was sitting in his olive-green recliner in the living room watching the news when we walked in. Mom stopped to talk as I made a mad dash for the stairs. Before locking myself in my bedroom for the night, I tiptoed into Mom and Dad's bathroom. I'd been hiding the goodie bag under my shirt, and I needed a safe place to stash it.

I hope I don't need this for a long time, I thought as I searched for a perfect hiding place. Inside Mom and Dad's small bathroom, there was a linen closet with a stack of old, raggedy towels that rarely got used. I put the bag behind them hoping that if Dad and Andy did find it, they'd assume it was Mom's.

"Good night," I yelled down the stairs to my parents,

who were having a hushed conversation under the sound of the TV. I assumed Mom was filling in Dad about what we'd just experienced. Oh brother, it was going to be weird around him too.

"Good night," they replied in unison.

I closed my door, got into my pajamas, and climbed into bed. I didn't want to think about the video, but I couldn't help it.

When I get older, I'm going to make eggs and then bleed every month.

Great. The mere thought of blood terrified me. From what I'd seen and experienced so far in life, blood meant crime scenes and accidents—never good things.

Blood running down the side of the white bathtub was why I'd been rushed to the hospital for stitches. It was also what had put Andy in the ER multiple times. I'd seen a lot of blood on Andy's feet after his clubfoot surgeries. I would never forget peeking into his bedroom and seeing bloody bandages hanging from his feet.

I'd also been schooled at church that Jesus shed his blood because of our sins, the worst of the worst. Blood always seemed to bring death, destruction, or dying.

I didn't yet understand all the ins and outs of puberty, but I did gather that periods only happened to girls, which made growing up as a girl even more frustrating. I didn't know what the boys had to deal with, if anything, but surely it wasn't as bad as monthly *bleeding*! Andy was so lucky! And I was so bummed. We had finally reached the point where we tolerated each other. I even saw Andy as my equal. Although he still annoyed me and we were very different, we were also the same in many ways. Plus, he was a great playmate. But puberty—it was going to threaten everything. It would suck all the fun out of life (or so I thought). Unfortunately, there was only one way to find out: go through it.

2

Changes

SHAVING LEGS AND ARMPITS, USING deodorant, wearing bras, buying bigger sizes, and dealing with hormones—so many changes. I soon realized these things came hard and fast with puberty. My female body was preprogrammed to morph. Ugh.

Some of the fourth-grade girls appeared to love the idea of puberty and other womanly stuff. They giggled and smiled at the subject. I wasn't one of them, which wasn't surprising. Keeping my distance from puberty went far deeper than feeling disappointed my body never consulted me about its upcoming changes. For starters, our church's emphasis on modesty carried not-so-subtle judgments against *those* women, the ones who loved lipstick more than the Lord. Scared to be like them, I separated myself from most feminine things by playing sports and calling myself a tomboy. Plus, I'd never acted very girly. I rejected dolls and Barbies, and I didn't much care for the color pink. Andy's Teenage Mutant Ninja Turtles and Power Rangers shows were *way* more interesting.

I'd started playing softball in second grade, which was okay. But truthfully, I liked the drinks and snacks in the cooler after games the best. I didn't appreciate the harsh dad who coached us, nor did I enjoy running around in the dirt. When my parents signed me up for basketball in fourth grade, it surprised all of us when I actually showed some skill.

"You've got a brother!" Mom pointed out after each one of my aggressive attempts to steal the ball, assuming Andy and my wrestling matches at home had toughened me up. Some very talented players who would go on to win our state championship in high school were on my team. Even as we learned the basics such as passing and dribbling, our games were full of energy, and our parents cheered madly. We dazzled all who watched us with our signature move: one of us would rebound the ball and bomb-lob it all the way downcourt near the basket. An open teammate would grab it for a lay-up and score. We'd eventually find out we didn't invent the play—other teams used cherry picking too.

"Wa*hoo*! Oh yeah! Good game! Great job!"

It felt awesome to receive compliments, pats on the back, and high fives. I enjoyed playing basketball so much, I couldn't imagine liking another sport more. But when I stepped onto the volleyball court, it surprised me too. I didn't just like volleyball; it became a sport I adored.

"Nice hit, Danielle-r!"

Coach D and the nickname she gave me should probably get most of the credit for my love of volleyball, as well as friends such as Leah. From the moment I learned how to serve aggressively and successfully, I was hooked. The game brought out the same athleticism as basketball, yet even more confidence. Nothing had ever felt so amazing—I could strategically hit over the net, and my opponents struggled to return my spikes and serves. The volleyball court surprisingly felt like a second home.

Although I'd always been a reserved kid who wrote plays and stories in her bedroom, sports woke up an inner strength. With white, square kneepads of armor affixed to my knees or a bouncy basketball in my hands, I felt the most like me.

Competition helped me overcome feeling shy. Teams introduced me to new friends. Games taught me how to talk to them. Sports weren't only fun to play, but over time, they helped me overcome the fear of being . . . a girl.

It was a fear I'd picked up one unfortunate day in kindergarten. A classmate chose to crawl under our table and look up my friend's skirt instead of doing his spelling worksheet. I didn't notice him at first, but immediately I sensed someone near our feet. Crawling around on his hands and knees, the boy had a slimy smirk on his face. Although we were all only five or six years old, I quickly understood what he had just done. He'd gotten a peek at her underwear.

"He-he-he," he snickered as he slid back into his seat.

His warning wasn't enough punishment, in my opinion. He'd violated not only my friend, but also me. Being the witness to his inappropriate peeking led me to write off dresses until junior high. I swore no boy would ever do that to me. With the exception of a couple of Christmas Days and Easter Sundays, I refused to wear anything with a skirt. My parents compromised and bought me dress pants for church. The pantsuits helped, but they couldn't undo what my classmate had taught me: being feminine was vulnerable. Girls were a target, especially those who wore dresses, makeup, and accessories.

Fortunately, as an athlete, I got away with ponytails, baggy T-shirts, and gym shorts. Sporty, rather than girly, became my signature look. But as puberty got closer, it wasn't exactly relenting. Not only did it refuse to compromise, it brought several new things, *girly* things, that absolutely rattled me. Things I couldn't avoid.

My body went from girlish to womanly nearly overnight. While sitting in a pew at my grandpa's funeral, of all places, I looked down and noticed dark, vining leg hair. It was a rare occasion—I was wearing a skirt. I despised them for good reasons. I tried to cross my legs to cover up, but there was no hiding. Mom noticed it too, and the next day, I had a puff of pink foaming cream in one hand, my own razor in the other, and a lesson on shaving as I sat on the edge of the bathtub.

But my legs weren't the only body part going through dramatic changes. My face kept getting peppered with red spots I was told not to pop (but couldn't help it). Although I wasn't battling major acne compared to friends at school, zits and breakouts came crashing into my world. Face wash appeared on the bathroom counter one day. Deodorant for teens too. Within a few months into fifth grade, just as I was turning eleven, I'd gone from little girl to adolescent young lady. A plethora of new womanly products began creating a bridge from girl to woman, but few items marked the path more than a bra.

I'd insisted my chest was flat, that I didn't need a bra, for a long time. In fourth grade after the video, Mom suggested buying me one, but I quickly declined her offer. Yet by fifth grade, my body was changing against my will, and my chest was getting bumpy.

Tomboys didn't wear bras. Girly girls did. I wanted nothing to do with them, especially after several girls in my grade started wearing them to school and showing them off. They'd find a way for the straps to "accidentally" peek out, or they'd wear bright colors under white shirts. As far as I could tell, they didn't actually *need* the bras yet, which made me despise wearing one even more. I did.

At first, I thought about ways to conceal my slowly growing chest without using a bra. Watching Roberta in *Now and Then* wrap her chest in duct tape gave me one idea, but that looked painful, and I didn't know where my dad kept his tape in the garage. I decided baggy T-shirts on warm days and puffy sweatshirts on cold days covered me up well enough. But one day, I outgrew my plan.

"We're going to the mall to find you a bra," Mom whispered one Saturday morning, leaving no room for a protest. She knew what my response would be, so she didn't ask for feedback.

As I plopped into the front seat of our car, I felt very perplexed. I didn't want to go shopping; yet at the same time, deep down inside, a tiny piece of me didn't mind it. Our family tended to be on the lower end of the middle class, so we didn't shop at the mall for new clothes very often. A trip to the department store was a treat. I was used to finding new shirts and pants while digging through black trash bags full of my cousin Kristi's hand-me-downs. To buy something new felt special. I just wished it wasn't *under*wear.

The drive to the mall was quiet, similar to other times Mom and I found ourselves alone in the car. I didn't know how to explain why I felt so nervous about wearing a bra and why I didn't want one. I assumed she made the connection. Wearing a bra was like wearing a dress. It would make me girly, uncomfortable, and, most importantly, vulnerable. Tomboys didn't like this stuff.

We found a parking spot and entered the department store through revolving doors. We quickly found ourselves in a perfume-saturated room with bright lights and tall displays of necklaces, face powders, and shoes. The tween section wasn't only marked by signs with arrows, but with posters of models my age. The models were the epitome of everything I wasn't—cute and pretty, fashionable and frilly. The perplexed feeling from the car came right back because I felt ashamed I didn't look more like them yet hopeful that maybe I could.

What's happening *to me?* I wasn't sure how to feel, but as conflict and confusion brewed, I decided to stick with disinterested. It was easier to stay sour and act hesitant. Had we gone shopping for cute outfits, or even out for a fun spa day, my attitude might have changed. But unfortunately, we were there for one reason. I knew better than to ask for anything else. I doubted we had the money.

"What about this one?"

Lost in a drowning sea of models posed on over-sized posters, I'd not noticed Mom. She'd already found the underwear section and begun searching for what I needed. At the sound of her voice, I looked up and saw two colorful triangles dangling high in the air off a hanger. Immediately my face turned red. I was mad and mortified. I had no doubt nearly everyone else in the store had heard her.

"Hmmm—mmmm," I grunted, using no words and my shaking head to fashion a negative response. Ducking so nobody could see me, I hid myself behind a six-pack of girls' briefs. Shopping for the bra was bad enough. If someone I knew saw us, I would die.

Mom eventually hung the triangles back on the rack and continued foraging.

My heart was racing, and my throat felt hot. I couldn't think of another time I'd felt so embarrassed. I knew bras were normal, but few of my friends at school wore them. I didn't want to be the first. I was ready to go home.

"How about this?"

I looked up and saw another vibrant option dangling from a hanger. It felt like she was in broadcasting.

"No . . . that won't work," I whispered, which clearly sparked frustration. A mom look came my way, and without any words, I knew my time was up. A standoff in the underwear section was not part of the day's plans. I finally gave in and cooperated.

"Only white—nothing colored or with prints. Look for a sports one."

I couldn't say the word "bra," but she knew what I

meant. If I had to wear one, it needed to be hidden—nothing any immature boys could see. She returned to the rack and found a few more options.

"Let's see if this fits."

Before I could scream "No!" she came at me with a bra, attempting to press it against my chest and measure.

I froze and then jumped back. "I'm sure it's fine. Let's go."

She'd gone too far, and I wanted to believe she knew it. Just about everyone in the store could tell I was unhappy. Although I was mad, once we got home, I realized she probably had no clue about what I feared awaited me at school. A few days later, my classmates proved me right. Although the bra was white, I couldn't totally hide it.

"Look, she's wearing a bra!" Both the boys and girls whispered in class.

It got even worse during recess when someone snuck behind me, and I felt a sharp sting race across my back.

Snap!

Laughter and the sound of tennis shoes sprinting across the playground behind me followed. To this day, I try to remind myself that my classmate didn't mean to *break* the bra itself, causing the small metal hook to fall down my back and into the top of my pants. I also think the incident made Mom aware of why I'd resisted wearing a bra for so long. She quickly made a second trip to the store to buy a replacement. It would be the first of many store runs she'd make to get me personal items.

I didn't know it right away. It was only after I stumbled to the hallway bathroom after getting out of bed that I realized something had changed overnight. The small dot of bright-red blood scared me at first and made my sleepy eyes shoot open.

Panic ran from my head to my toes, but I quickly realized what was happening. Memories from the video flooded in, and I was thankful, for once, for the hidden goodie bag. I tiptoed out of the hallway bathroom, grabbed a change of clothes from my bedroom, and slipped into my parents' bathroom.

"I'm glad I kept this . . ." I admitted to myself as I quietly unzipped the bag, careful to go slowly so nobody would hear and wonder what I was doing. I thumbed through the brochures and tampons until I found a thick, white maxi pad. It was wrapped up like a puffy cloud, yet less heavenly. Holding it ever so gently in my hands, I unwrapped each side silently, in slow motion.

Although I was aware of pads and tampons, I didn't know how to use them, and I'd certainly not been open to a discussion or lesson. Assuming I was experiencing a moment nearly all women faced, I decided to figure it out. I refused to call for help.

The illustrations printed on the wrapper didn't indicate which way was up or down, so I guessed. I assumed that feeling like a bulky, uncomfortable diaper was stuck between my legs meant I'd done it right. I wrapped up all the trash in toilet paper and carefully buried it at the bottom of the trash can.

For the rest of the morning, I followed my normal routine. I got dressed, brushed my teeth, and combed my hair before sitting across from Andy at the kitchen table to eat a bowl of cereal. I stuffed an extra pad deep into my backpack and planned to tell Mom about my period later that night. But with each bite of cereal, I started to feel guilty. The pad was really uncomfortable, a constant reminder of my hidden news. By the time Andy finished eating and left the kitchen, I'd changed my mind.

"Um . . . I got my period today."

Mom had walked through the kitchen, and with both Dad and Andy upstairs, it was perfect timing. I delivered my news in the most unemotional and quiet way. Fortunately, she handled it sensitively.

"Do you have everything you need?" she whispered back, careful to not speak too loudly. This was different. I couldn't tell how she felt—sad or excited.

"Yes—I've got pads from the goodie bag they gave us at school last year."

"I'll go to the store and get you other supplies, less bulky ones, after work."

I wasn't sure how she knew the pad was so gigantic. Maybe I'd not hidden the goodie bag as well as I thought, but I felt relieved to hear there were thinner options. Thank God.

I eventually made it to school and experienced a new day. A new era. I was a new person living in a shell from my old life. Although I'd boarded the same yellow school bus, the seat felt different. I walked into the same classroom, surrounded by my same friends, yet suddenly they didn't know everything about me. At recess, I didn't join the basketball game like the day before. I didn't feel comfortable running up and down the court with a puffy cloud between my legs. Like a visitor in my own world, I tried to grasp my new normal, life with a monthly period. I thought about it constantly, at least at first.

Is this pad going to leak? I can't change it at school; people will hear! Can people tell I've gotten my period?

I didn't have to ask around. I knew. Like the bra, I was one of the first girls in my grade, and definitely the first girl in my group of friends, to start. I wished I could have held my period off longer, but my body didn't listen. Alone and embarrassed, I did everything possible to hide it. We kept all the pads in Mom's bathroom so Andy and my friends wouldn't find them in the hallway. On the weeks my period came, I wore two layers of underwear, under my volleyball shorts, under my jeans to avoid any leaks at school. I refused to change pads (and tampons once I got brave enough to try them) in public bathrooms. I kept a jacket with me and tied it around my waist for extra safety. Despite my best efforts to hide the fact I was on my period, I wasn't always successful. Leaks led to some of the worst days of my life, even more embarrassing than bra shopping.

The sight of blood grossed me out, and I couldn't get used to it. Although my doctor said getting my period was a sign of good health at my yearly physical, it didn't feel healthy. It felt horrible.

Cramps hurt my abdomen, and the anxiety of dealing with

Like a visitor in my own world, I tried to grasp my new normal, life with a monthly period.

blood once a month overwhelmed me. But over time, I learned the video was right. All girls go through puberty.

Although dealing with a period made my life harder, it got easier when my friends started getting theirs too. They were more open than I was, but I'd often chime in with "me too" when they'd share. By sixth grade, I wasn't the only one shaving my legs, wearing bras, and dealing with "that time of the month." Plus, I found some guides who seemed to understand what puberty felt like and could help me through it. Guides who seemed to know me better than I knew myself and understood what my heart desired.

3

Salads and Suntans

"READY TO PAINT OUR NAILS?" my cousin Kristi asked as we ran through the crowded room, careful to not knock into any family members squeezed into Grandma Pat and Grandpa Dorman's house. Although we had a big family, Pat and Dorman had raised four kids who all married and had more kids, and we all insisted on getting together in their small ranch house in northern Missouri each holiday. Without it, it wouldn't have felt like Christmas.

A lot of my other cousins loved Christmas at Grandma Pat's for the presents and family gift exchange, and Dad liked it because he got to see his family. I'd always enjoyed Grandma Pat and her house because she hosted me, by myself, for a week-long getaway during several summers. I craved alone time with her. But at age twelve, I loved her house for one reason: my cousin Kristi.

Unlike me, Kristi wasn't stuck in elementary school. She had gone on to junior high and then high school. Being three years older, she was well-versed in the world of all things teenage. While she could have kept me out of her life, as I was an annoying tween cousin, she shared every detail.

Since as long as I could remember, I loved being with Kristi. Our connection went far back. Some of my grandparents' earliest photos of their grandkids displayed on the wall showed me, Kristi, and her older sister in matching outfits. It was just us girls until Andy showed up one year later. I didn't remember the memories of playing with Kristi as infants, but I did recall weekends we'd travel to her house as a young kid. Her family moved a lot, and we often took car trips to visit them. Over the course of my life, I'd travel across Iowa, Missouri, and Nebraska state lines to see her. Andy loved to go too, since she had a little brother. Their house was a destination vacation spot for us. I loved it when her mom, my Aunt Deb, called me her third daughter. Their house was a safe place to have fun.

Since Kristi's mom and dad, like my parents, ran a conservative Christian home, we had similar rules. In fact, my mom looked to Aunt Deb's parameters as a guide for me and Andy. I was often told: "What goes for Kristi is the same for you" when it came to boys, music, makeup, and clothing.

Sifting through trash bags of Kristi's hand-me-downs was like finding pure gold. I knew if she got to wear something, I could wear it too. It's likely that I took to sports so much because Kristi played softball, basketball, and volleyball. She also called herself a tomboy. In every way, I wanted to be like her—except I kept my favorite color green (not purple), and my favorite animal remained the elephant, not the dolphin.

Kristi was older and cool. Although I often didn't feel like I fit in with other girls, I fit with her. It was comforting, especially as my body began changing, because she was also going through puberty. It made figuring out how to be tomboys, yet also embracing womanhood, a little easier when we did it together.

Despite being in a packed house with one bathroom (not counting the small closet that had been remodeled to offer our large family a second toilet, sink, and mirror), Kristi and I had our routine. Toward the end of the evening, once the tables were cleared and the dishes got washed, the adults sat in the living room to visit. Our younger cousins scattered to watch TV and play with toys in what was nicknamed the Pretend Room. But Kristi and I had outgrown it, so we darted to the bathroom. We'd dig through Grandma's basketful of pink and red nail polish bottles and sit on the white tile floor to paint our toenails. It was the highlight of my trip, and oftentimes, the whole holiday. Christmas was less about the gifts I opened. I relished the time spent with Kristi more than anything.

"Time for magazines?"

Once our nail polish dried and no longer felt sticky, we'd move to the corner of the living room near Grandma Pat's wooden magazine rack, which was always stuffed with at least six to twelve months of different magazines, full and overflowing. I wasn't sure if Grandma didn't like

The magazines were a one-stop place to learn how to act and look like a perfect woman.

to clean it out, or if she'd saved them on purpose for family gatherings. The rack sat next to the arm of the pastel plaid couch and the wooden curio cabinet that held Precious Moments figurines. We stayed quiet as we got out and started flipping past each glossy cover.

For a Christian woman married to a devout deacon, my grandma surprisingly subscribed to a lot of worldly magazines. But we weren't complaining. We loved reading the advice offered to modern-day housewives. Although the articles and ads clearly weren't for girls our age, they were sooo appealing. Kristi and I loved thumbing through the slick pages for tips on everything we needed to know as young women.

We'd lie on our tummies pressed against the soft carpet and, page after page, take in ideas. We learned about cooking the ideal supper and folding a fitted sheet. (Who knew I wasn't the only one who couldn't do it?) Thanks to articles and pictures, we'd understand how to file our fingernails, correctly use shampoo, buy the right clothes for our body shapes, and choose the best creams for our skin. I even recall a step-by-step illustration showing how to use living room furniture as exercise equipment.

The magazines were a one-stop place to learn how to act and look like a perfect woman. If the beauty articles didn't tell us what to do and use, the ads did. From the housekeeping magazines to those focused on weight loss and family, there was one common theme. All the models had rosy cheeks, shadowy eyes, bronze skin, and slender bodies.

"Oh wow, I want hair like that!" we'd remark while swooning over shampoo ads. "Whoa, look at his six-pack abs!" "Her outfit is so cute. I love that skirt and those shoes!"

The once-proclaimed tomboys disappeared as the allure of feeling beautiful felt stronger. Like pirates searching for priceless treasure, we pored over the magazines as maps. While the family members surrounding us taught us their preferred path for life, one that focused on church and God stuff, the magazines taught us other things—ways to look pretty and attract guys. It didn't take long for me to realize I needed to make a lot of changes.

"Danielle, if this doesn't stop, I'm calling your parents."

I really didn't think a little salad in the trash was a big deal, but the look on my school counselor's face said it all, and her stern words backed it up.

I'd always known my counselor as a nice, friendly lady who cut her blond hair in a short pixie style. She hadn't changed it after four years of my knowing her, which was comforting—especially as I hit fifth and sixth grades. In a time of life when everything else seemed to shift drastically, things that stayed the same brought comfort. The counselor's hairstyle was the same year after year, but her new tone with me was different.

While flipping through the magazines, I'd noticed all the models looked skinny, and I'd returned home inspired. I looked different from them, and not just because they were older. Compared to their tall and skinny bodies, I looked short and stubby. I knew I wasn't fat, but my stomach looked puffy to me. It wasn't hard and firm with defined muscles. To look like the models would require changes.

Puberty had taught me that when it came to my body, a lot was out of my control. It hadn't asked for my permission to grow, and it made me uncomfortable when it did. While I couldn't help it that my chest was growing shapelier or that my widening caused me to need new jeans, I could control what I ate and how skinny my stomach looked, or so I thought. I decided to try.

The weight-loss magazines offered plenty of help. But a made-for-TV movie about an actress who struggled with anorexia gave me more ideas (unfortunately backfiring on the point of the movie). As I watched scenes where she hid food in her bedroom and overexercised to look skinny, I secretly thought, *She looks good. I want that too.*

She lied about eating, and in the end, she got really sick. But that part didn't scare me. I was fixated on how she managed to get to zero fat and make her collarbone protrude from her oversized sweatshirts. Although I couldn't do everything she did, I mulled over a few of her sly ways. Eating *nothing* wasn't an option for me, because of our family dinners.

"Why aren't you eating? Here, have some bread and butter." I could just hear my parents during dinner. Like most suburban families, many weeknights were spent at sports practice, piano lessons, or church programs. Yet we did manage to eat together as a family many nights of the week, even if we sat around the table for a few minutes. I could only imagine what my parents would say if I sat at the table and refused to eat everything.

"Are you sick? You have to eat something!"

Not eating wasn't an option, but neither was binge-ing. I couldn't stand the thought of making myself puke. Yet food was a key to body size and shape. Fortunately, another creative idea came: Eat everything but dinner.

It was genius. I wouldn't be lying if asked, "Are you eating?" but I'd eat just enough to get by. Eating very little food was surely a way to get skinny—I couldn't wait to try.

I decided to experiment with breakfast. I'd never loved the first meal of the day, but Mom insisted I eat before school. She'd eventually compromised, and instead of expecting me to force down cereal, Andy's favorite food, she started buying me grab-and-go foods.

"I've got a toaster strudel and apple!" I'd yell before heading to the bus stop. And that was the truth—the breakfast items were in my hands. But on the way to the stop, I walked over to the street's storm drain, looked left and right, and then chucked both the wrapped pastry and fresh fruit. Way ahead of me, Andy never noticed.

"Goodbye, breakfast." I laughed as the silver package disappeared into the darkness to, I assumed, feed the rats or something. It felt so awesome to be in control, I repeated it the next morning. By the end of the week, unbeknownst to Mom, an entire box of wrapped pastries and a week's worth of apples were rotting at the bottom of the drain. My experiment was working so well, I set my sights on lunch.

Similar to our family dinners, skipping lunch altogether wasn't an option. But I could request a chef's salad. It was a special perk for sixth graders, which I appreciated (although I didn't exactly care for the taste of lettuce and carrots).

I remembered reading an article about how eating salads can make you skinny, and I'd watched Mom and her friends turn to vegetables when they wanted to lose weight. I'd been told "Eat your fruits and veggies!" all my life. Ordering a bowl of lettuce for lunch wouldn't cause any problems. Nobody needed to know the only reason I got it: throw it all away.

The first day I planned to skip lunch was harder than I anticipated. The smells of cheese pizza and chicken-fried steak wafting from my friends' trays taunted me, and truth be told, I was hungry. I was used to skipping one meal, but not two. I found myself sitting at a lunch table with friends who didn't get it. Although several wore bras and had gotten their periods, their bodies were still girlish and skinny. They weren't getting curvy like mine. I assumed they wouldn't understand my eating plan, so I didn't mention it. I also didn't expect them to notice or watch me.

At first, my plan went perfectly. Like a rabbit, I nibbled on a few pieces of lettuce, and once the aides called out "Pick up your trays and form a line," I'd dump the bowl in the trash.

But a week or so after I began dumping salads, the counselor pulled me aside. "I hear you're throwing your lunch in the trash. This can be a sign of something serious, like eating disorders." And then she threatened to call my parents.

My heart sank. I was Mom's Angel Face. I hated disappointing adults, and the feeling of getting caught was the worst. Who told her? Had she been watching? My questions never got answered, but I angrily assumed my friends had ratted me out. Over time, I softened up and realized they'd helped save me. And I began ordering pizza again.

I took the counselor's warning to heart and could see why she'd pulled me aside. I had many of the major warning signs of an eating disorder. I became thankful she gave me a second chance to prove I'd start eating again before calling home. I knew in some cases, girls with eating disorders couldn't help it, and they needed treatment. I'd not quite reached that point—nor did I want to.

Although I did start eating three meals a day, plus snacks, again, I still wanted to look and feel skinny. Tomboy or not, I wanted to be a hot girl turning boys' heads. I wanted to feel as beautiful as the models in the magazines. But I wasn't going to get there riding the waves of an eating disorder, I realized. Fortunately, to slim down, the magazines suggested several more ways.

Maybe Mom and her friends got their advice from magazines too. I wasn't sure, but I did begin to notice that most females carried the universal desire to feel skinny and look pretty. I was the only one (that I knew of) who tried cutting out food, but I certainly wasn't the only female striving for a slender, flawless body. She'd always looked skinny to me, but Mom and her friends (sometimes even Dad) went on special diets and eating plans when they wanted to lose weight. In addition to cutting out sugar and buying more vegetables, Mom exercised.

It was common to see her pedaling on our stationary bike, walking the treadmill, or following a silly workout tape. Usually I sat on the couch and laughed. But puberty was changing me. One day, instead of teasing her from the couch, I asked to join. *Sweatin' to the Oldies* looked like a lot of fun.

"Sure, come on!"

Out of all her low-impact aerobics tapes, Richard Simmons was by far my favorite. I loved his bright-red striped shorts and curly hair. The music was fun and upbeat. The crazy man's energy was downright contagious. I didn't mind that the people working out behind him were way older than me. I gladly, joyfully followed along as we hopped, stepped, clapped, and did arm circles in the middle of our living room.

Basketball and volleyball practice kept me active, but the tapes helped me exercise even more. I was motivated to slim down. Junior high was getting closer. Each day when the school bus drove past the junior high, I felt both anxiety and hope that I'd somehow fit in. I knew the hallways would be full of other girls who'd gone through puberty, but I assumed that just like in the magazines, most of them would look prettier. The tomboy in me didn't care; the woman growing up inside of me did. But I wasn't quite a woman yet, and I didn't understand that slimming down and changing a body (the healthy way) takes time.

After our living room workouts, I'd run upstairs to wipe off my sweat and check my progress. I expected to see results within hours, or at maximum, a few days. Lifting up the hem of my T-shirt, I'd search for muscle lines and signs of a flatter stomach. But unfortunately, the hoped-for progress never came. The same white, puffy stomach I'd seen all my life stared back at me.

I knew I wasn't technically fat, but my stomach looked fat to me. It certainly wasn't model skinny, nor was it washboard-abs strong.

Sighing in defeat, I couldn't help but feel disappointed. Exercise and eating healthy were the two biggies. Did the magazines lie? Or were the tips only for older women? I wasn't sure if I had the patience, or the time, to find out. My body was already blooming. If I wanted to survive junior high and have any hope in high school, I needed to find another way to get beautiful—and quickly.

Makeup was another option, but just like Kristi, I couldn't wear it until I turned thirteen. I assumed we didn't have the money to buy new clothes from the mall, and while I actually liked my long, dark hair, it was pretty plain. But one day on summer break, my neighborhood friend Sarah had a brilliant idea. "Want to tan on my driveway?"

My eyes lit up—it was perfect. Tanning had never crossed my mind, although come to think of it, magazine models were bronze, not white and freckled like me.

"YES!" It was a no-brainer reply. I could think of no better way to spend a hot summer afternoon.

Home alone, we grabbed a snack and drink from the kitchen before heading to the bathroom to rummage through her mom's totes. My eyes lit up as Sarah pulled out a dark-brown bottle with streams of oil dripping down its side.

I read the label aloud. "One hundred percent suntan lotion."

A faint smell of coconut filled the bathroom as we cracked it open. We grabbed two colorful beach towels and ran downstairs, through the garage, and into the ninety-degree day. It was perfect. Sarah grabbed the oily bottle first to demonstrate how to spread it evenly. I needed the guidance; we had nothing like this at our house. Mom and I didn't have the red hair, but thanks to our Irish ancestors, we did get their fair skin tone. The only lotions we stocked up on were big bottles of SPF 70.

I took the oily bottle from Sarah and carefully followed her steps. Once we lathered up, we shook out our towels, spread them flat onto the hot concrete driveway, and lay down.

I'm actually doing it—no more pasty white legs for me! I thought as I shielded my eyes from the bright sun and caught a whiff of the coconut-scented oil. Full of hope that tanning would make me beautiful, I had another thought. *Who am I?* I wasn't quite sure anymore.

I was still a tomboy playing on several sports teams and going to summer camps to improve my skills. But I was also a tween girl waking up to a changing body every morning with new thoughts and feelings. I was becoming a new person, my own person, someone different from the rest of my family. I wasn't sure how to express it yet, but for starters, I was going to be tan.

"Let's check for our lines!"

I'd followed Sarah's lead and flipped from front to back a few times. Clueless about how much time tanning took, I eagerly raced with her back through the garage, up the stairs, and into the bathroom. We flipped on the lights to study ourselves in the mirror.

"You go first!" I insisted, mostly because I still wasn't sure what to do.

We'd tanned in our clothes, not our swimsuits, mostly because mine was at home. Rolled shorts and tucked shirts became the litmus test of our success. Sarah went first by rolling her shorts a little higher. We both squealed when we saw it—a perfect tan line.

"It worked! And fast!" I said, excited and giddy for her.

Next it was my turn. I did the exact same thing. Standing at the mirror, I hiked up my shorts a little higher in hopes of revealing a similar line. Nothing but red marks from where my shorts squeezed my thighs and a couple of new freckles showed up. I tried again by rolling my shorts higher, but no tan line ever came. Bummer.

An arrow of disappointment shot through my heart.

Pasty white wasn't beautiful; it looked nothing like what I saw on TV or in the magazines. When I'd stand and face myself in the mirror, I saw nothing even remotely pretty.

Beauty just wasn't for me. Upset and embarrassed, I went home. I didn't want Sarah to feel bad, but I was so sad and unhappy. I spent the rest of the afternoon and evening in my bedroom, trying to hide from Mom what had happened. By dinnertime, it was obvious. My skin had gone from light pink to lobster red. Our bottles of SPF 70 and green aloe vera looked like a goldmine.

The sunburn was so bad, it hurt to move. Yet it hurt the small amounts of self-esteem I carried even more.

Pasty white wasn't beautiful; it looked nothing like what I saw on TV or in the magazines. When I'd stand and face myself in the mirror, I saw nothing even remotely pretty.

My body refused to cooperate. I just didn't get it. First, it was puberty's unfortunate timing as it brought boobs to a tomboy and periods before anyone else my age. My clothing sizes kept going up no matter how much I exercised, and my puffy stomach wouldn't flatten. I tried to get skinny. I wanted to look pretty. But it was hopeless. Nothing worked. The confidence I'd once found on the volleyball court was gone; my hope had totally faded. But fortunately, not for long.

4

Camp Shamineau

"**F**INALLY."

It was all I could whisper. It was all I could think as I found a window seat on the chartered bus and waved goodbye through the window to Mom and Dad. I could barely see them waving back from the church parking lot, beneath the yellowed streetlight that was too dim to light the dark night.

Just minutes before, I'd bounded several tall metal stairs and boarded the bus that planned to drive throughout the night and take our youth group to camp in northern Minnesota. The other students on the bus were giddy-excited. It sounded like a school gymnasium before an all-school assembly; their laughs and loud talk made it nearly impossible to hear.

I shuffled down the aisle looking left and right and found an empty row toward the middle of the bus on the left side. The seats were upholstered in a velvety blue fabric that felt soft to touch as I slid into the seat closest to the window. I pressed my nose against it and squinted to make out my family standing outside in the dusk. Once they saw me, we waved at each other, and I sat back. A mixture of relief and fear hit all at once.

Getting away from home for a whole week felt like breaking free. Outside of the weeks I spent at Grandma Pat's house without my brother, I was almost always at our house. We didn't vacation much other than out-of-town family visits. Usually life was spent in the suburbs. I welcomed the chance to go somewhere new, especially without Mom, Dad, or Andy. Dealing with a surge of hormones and a plethora of new things was hard enough as a tween. Mom and Dad weren't making it any easier.

I didn't know how to explain it, nor did I dare mention it to anyone. Revealing the tension would have ruined our family's squeaky-clean reputation. I knew better. But things at home were tense. Mom seemed really unhappy. In starting up his own business, Dad needed to move two hours away for training over the course of nine months. The night we moved him into his apartment, I cried and cried. Although he came home every weekend, I didn't like life without him. Forever a daddy's girl, it wasn't the same at home. Mom managed to corral Andy and me, and our summertime rhythm of picking up the house before going to the swimming pool all day was fun. I assumed Dad would join our rhythm once he moved back home. But that wasn't the case.

He did move home, and we all pitched in to get the business going, but instead of it being over-the-top happy, things felt weird between Mom and Dad. We didn't talk about the tension much, at least as a family, but I could sense it was constantly there. At the dinner table. At church. Something between the two of them felt off. But my whole life felt off with junior high just about to begin. A week at camp sounded nice. Even if it was about God.

For all my life, attending church was never an option. We didn't just go every Sunday morning, we went Sunday and Wednesday nights too. Making colorful beaded necklaces during Vacation Bible School, singing with Psalty the Singing Songbook, and sitting through VeggieTales movies was the backdrop of my childhood. I didn't mind it at first, yet in midst of puberty, I became aware of popularity, and I realized most of the cool kids at school and in the neighborhood didn't go to church. My forced attendance soon felt daunting. Being one of the only girls my age made it harder to go. Once I got my period, I hoped for a special invitation to join the youth group early, but it never came. Stuck with a bunch of little kids in a choir room, one night it got even worse. Our leaders cast me as the lead female in our upcoming children's program. Mortified, I couldn't say no.

So months later, I took the stage to play the part—a basketball player who set a good Christian example at her school. After the bow, I walked away humiliated and promised myself I'd never attend church once it became my choice. I could just imagine the chuckles coming from students in the youth group who sat in the back pews of the dark sanctuary. The thought of them watching me act alongside the kids made my stomach cramp.

I hated church just as much as I hated my body, although nobody I passed in the church hallways would have known. The desire to please overcame the temptation to rebel.

Yet if I had to attend church, which I did, I wanted to be with the youth group. They had their own modular building and taped posters of Christian bands to the walls. I often heard loud rock music coming from big speakers and watched students come and go. Plus, the youth leaders, Nick and Leslie, seemed cool. They became even cooler when they extended an invitation to camp before I officially started junior high. Even if camp was going to talk about God a lot, I was willing to give it a try. Not expecting to enjoy it or to quickly make friends on the bus, I was surprised.

"Hey! Can I sit with you?"

It was the face of someone I distantly recognized.

"It's me—Jordan. Remember? Our parents are friends."

It took me a few seconds, but the memory of his face, and family, finally came. We'd been children the last time we'd seen each other. His hair wasn't as dark and wavy, and his voice hadn't been so deep. I became self-consciously aware I probably looked really different, too, although Jordan didn't seem repelled.

"Hey! Sure, you can sit here!" I quickly moved my pillow and backpack out of the way, surprised he wanted to sit by me but by no means disappointed.

"So you're in youth now?" he asked as a charming smile spread across his face.

"Yeah, I finally made it." I nervously laughed, hoping

he'd not witnessed me acting with little kids on the church stage. He didn't mention it and proceeded to shove his backpack under the seat. As he moved around, I smelled his . . . cologne? It was a manly fragrance, a pleasing scent compared to wafts of salty chips and candy bars already stinking up the bus.

The luggage compartment latches on the outside of the bus ker-chunked shut—it was time to go. Since I'd never ridden a chartered bus before, I was curious about what came next. And with a friend sitting next to me, and a handsome one at that, a new feeling floated in. I was actually *excited*—at church!

The bus pulled away slowly, and the dark parking lot vanished. Jordan and I returned to our conversation, rapidly catching each other up on ten years. We talked about everything—our neighborhoods, our friends, our parents. It was comforting to make an instant friend, and I didn't mind him being an older, taller guy one bit. I'd be lying if I said there wasn't an instant chemistry. But as we talked, I became aware that one, he had a girlfriend, and two, he was more like a big brother. With everything going on in my life, I needed a good friend.

I'd assumed the youth leaders would separate the junior high students from high schoolers. But my assumptions were wrong, as Jordan sat next to me—and stayed. I'd just finished sixth grade and he was headed to high school, yet nobody told him to move.

As the bus picked up speed on the highway and we zoomed past big signs, Jordan encouraged me to follow him into the aisle. "Come with me. I want to introduce you to some people."

I rose shyly, and he led me toward a big group gathered in the back of the bus, where his older brother Jared sat with his friends. I barely remembered Jared. He was several years older than I was, as were the juniors and seniors sitting around him. But that didn't stop Jordan from reintroducing me, first to his brother and then to everyone else. When they didn't ignore me or laugh about my young age, I was shocked.

"Hi, I'm Ryan."

"I'm Grace."

"Hey, I'm Kep."

"I'm Mike."

"I'm Dave."

"I'm Jennifer."

One by one, they introduced themselves, unfazed by my young age. And then they really shocked me. Scooting over, they patted an open space on the blue cushions so I could sit. Mind blown. They cared . . . about *me*? It was surreal. I plopped down between the older girls and got comfy.

The sights outside the windows kept transforming, and we appeared to be driving through both well-lit cities and abandoned areas studded with evergreen trees. Like the landscapes outside the window, I too was morphing. As the upperclassmen welcomed me into their inner circle, I felt the foreign feeling of acceptance. In an unexpected way, I *belonged* with them. It was especially nice to be the youngest . . . for once. I didn't know what was happening. I had no idea what to expect. I just needed to follow my leaders and the older students, who, fortunately, appeared to like me.

If this is what church is like with youth group, maybe it isn't so bad.

Eventually, I began feeling sleepy and returned to my seat, where I dozed off and on for a few hours until waking up at the sunrise. The dawn's shooting rays couched between pink and red hues made for a beautiful alarm clock. It was obvious we'd made it to Minnesota—the signs on the highway indicated we were close to Mall of America. Excited for our scheduled stop at one of the largest shopping malls in the world, I had no plans to relive past trips. I'd stay far away from all bras.

After a short stop for eating and shopping at Mall of America, our bus rolled back onto the highway. I rested my head against the big window and fell asleep again. When the bus came to a long stop accompanied by loud, squeaky brakes, I opened my eyes to the bright sun again. This time, huge evergreen trees, double the size of Christmas trees, surrounded us. A strong scent of summer pine rushed in. A gentle breeze hinted that a nearby lake was just past our view. Everything was so calm and peaceful. So serene.

"Welcome to Camp *Sham*ineau!" Nick hollered like a sports announcer. We filed out of the bus to get our instructions. I stretched my arms to both wake up and wave goodbye to my new, older friends while looking for the tween girls my age.

We made our way to our temporary home—a log cabin dorm with sturdy wooden bunk beds and a low-tech pull-string light that swung to and fro each time someone opened the door. I chose the bottom bunk just to the left and quickly made my bed and tacked a few pictures of my friends to the wall to help it feel more like home. Within minutes, the pungent smell of cucumber melon perfume billowed through the air.

We decided to tour the campgrounds before dinner and worship service. Following a camp guide up a wood chipped path, we arrived at our first stop: the girls' detached bathrooms.

This is perfect!

Before leaving for camp, I'd felt most anxious about two things: starting my period and pooping around other people.

I didn't want to experience either, so the detached bathrooms worked great. Should I need to go number two at night, sneaking out was easy. Mental note made. Our tour continued and culminated in the mess hall where we would eat. It was also where I learned the rumors were true—we could drink unlimited glasses of Coke with every meal. I was having fun and enjoying myself, grateful to be at camp. On my own, free from home, my heart was opening—and just in time for evening worship.

> Before leaving for camp, I'd felt most anxious about two things: starting my period and pooping around other people.

If I thought the charter bus was loud, the sanctuary took noise to an even higher level. A couple of youth leaders from Kansas City had designed the camp, which meant hundreds of students from other churches had also ridden throughout the night and guzzled unlimited Cokes before walking into the room. Laughing, yelling, shouting, and jumping around—it was typical teenage. I'd never seen anything like this at church.

The shy girl in me hesitated to enter the room, but fortunately, Jordan let me stay near him. Although happy to be there, I felt overwhelmed. Eventually, the overhead music lowered, and the room quieted as we found a row of open seats.

A guy named Billy with a long goatee stepped onstage with his acoustic guitar. "We're going to kick off tonight with a few worship songs."

Worship? With no organ, piano, or hymnal book? Nice!

Billy strummed songs I didn't know, but I caught on quickly. He even played an original song about God's amazing love and a king dying for me. Thanks to words projected onto the wall, I sang along (and actually enjoyed it). Once the music stopped, our youth ministers introduced the speaker, a guy named Voddie. He had the presence of a football player and the booming voice of a coach. Diving right in, Voddie began passionately preaching. At first I was afraid he was upset and yelling, but then I realized it was his sermon style. Eventually, I started listening.

"Make your faith your *own*—not your parents' faith."

He sounded serious. As his sermon went on, descriptions of a "lukewarm Christian" flowed. My heart beat quickly, and my seat grew hot. Had he been watching me at home? Sure, I believed in God and I attended church. I'd even been baptized with Andy before fourth grade. But clearly, I was not into the God scene. I hadn't expected that to change.

Sweat began to pool under my armpits, and I uncomfortably wiggled in my chair. I knew Voddie was talking to me, or about me, but I refused to look up—or worse, make eye contact. While concluding his sermon, Voddie issued a challenge. It was different from the traditional altar calls to which I'd grown calloused.

"If anyone's in this room and you want to confess you haven't been living out your faith—and you want to get your relationship right with God—stand up."

I froze, shocked the first night of camp was so strong. So bold.

No—I can't.

I knew I needed to stand. But I refused to draw attention to myself.

I've already done this. I prayed the Sinner's Prayer and got baptized. I'm good. I'll do better, I silently reasoned with myself.

Yet as the room went eerily quiet, my heart continued to beat profusely. Before I could comprehend what was happening, it was like someone lifted me from my sweaty armpits and stood me to my feet. An odd combination of peace and panic hit.

Did I just stand up, or was I picked up?

I wasn't exactly sure. Voddie began praying, and I closed my eyes, trying to simply breathe. Although I'd resisted standing, I did want to get right with God. An obsession over beauty had led to a warped body image. Embarrassed to be a Christian, I hid, sometimes lied about, my faith to friends. The God I knew was boring, yet the one Voddie preached about sounded exciting. He spoke of a faith, and supernatural power, I wanted . . . yet didn't quite have.

"Can our leaders come get these kids?"

I looked around and saw Leslie motioning for me to walk toward her.

"Why did you stand up tonight?"

We'd walked outside, into a cool, calm night, so we could talk alone. Smile calming with eyes twinkling, Leslie's question was not in the least threatening, and I let my guard down. "I guess I felt like that person he was describing tonight—I'm a lukewarm Christian— and I'm not sure what I believe about God."

I could get behind a God who actually cared about me and how I felt, not just a God expecting to see me in church every Sunday.

I began to share my honest feelings about church.

She seemed to understand without judging or making me feel bad. "God wants a relationship with us—a real back-and-forth relationship where we talk to Him and He talks to us."

Leslie's words sounded both familiar and foreign, a message I'd been taught my whole life. Yet somehow, I heard it differently. It made perfect sense. I could get behind a God who actually cared about me and how I felt, not just a God expecting to see me in church every Sunday. As we continued to talk, my chest pounding slowed, and my armpits dried. Leslie offered a tip: read the Bible each day.

Why am I just now learning about why we read the Bible and daily quiet times? I wondered. Genuinely confused, I thought the Bible was for memorizing verses and listing rules and commandments. Not once had I used it for something so personal. But I was open to trying.

"Thank you so much!" I said to Leslie before offering a hug and running off to find my friends.

Later that night, I thought about the sermon and everything Leslie had said. I prayed on my own without anyone telling me to. It was weird. I actually *wanted* to talk to God.

As camp went on, the girl who had boarded the bus with a hard heart, the one who had promised to never attend church as an adult, was softening—quickly.

Over the next few days, I found myself learning and singing more worship songs. Taking notes during sermons, I listened closely. The noes in my heart turned to yeses when Jesus and God came up. Every Bible verse I read sounded like a secret door leading to another secret door. Suddenly God was very real and very *in*teresting.

On the final night of camp, leaders warned us about "mountaintop experiences." They said it's easy to build a strong faith at camp but become lukewarm at home and school. But once I made it back to the suburbs, I experienced the opposite: being in Kansas City only fueled my faith more. Others could tell.

When Nick asked if I'd share what God had taught me at camp, my testimony, from the pulpit at church, I eagerly stepped onto the stage. I shared again a few nights later in youth group. Church wasn't the only place I was changing though. I was different at home too. When Mom asked for help or cooperation around the house, I didn't give her attitude. I was even nice to Andy, which at times felt like a miracle.

"You've come back from camp a different person," Mom commented one day after I squealed with excitement about going to youth group. In addition to staying close to Jordan after camp, I'd made new Christian friends. With them behind me, stepping into the front doors of junior high was a breeze.

Truth be told, I still didn't feel very beautiful. Nothing like a cover model. Yet my newfound faith helped me refocus. Pretty and popular—or not—God still cared about me. In fact, He was answering big prayers. For example, He'd helped my fears about going to the bathroom at camp. Not only did I not start my period that week, but I also didn't go number two at all.

5

Titanic

CRIMSON METAL LOCKERS SLAMMING SHUT. Squeaky sneakers echoing off concrete floors and tiled walls. A loud cafeteria with a distinct aroma: greasy french fries meet cardboard pepperoni pizza. There was so much about junior high that I'd heard about and expected, and most of what I envisioned came true. Everyone was right—it was way better than elementary school.

I'd felt the normal jitters before starting school, the flutters that come with anything new and different. The night before seventh grade, I didn't go to sleep easily. But I survived the first day, and to my surprise, it took only a few more for a new routine to feel familiar. While waking up at six thirty and walking from class to class weren't my favorites, I liked junior high's changes. Seventh grade meant freedom. Seventh grade meant I wasn't the only one with a growing female body.

Not only was I happy with school itself, I was thrilled

I'd heard of moms and dads not getting along and eventually getting divorced, but that was something that happened to other people, especially people who didn't go to church.

when several of my friends were in my classes, especially my best friend, Emily. We had become connected instantly in sixth grade when she enrolled in our school, and as fate would have it, she lived close enough for us to ride our bikes to each other's houses. And—we had the exact same bike! As we'd ride the streets together, the independence felt liberating. I was so glad to have her as a friend in junior high. Going through puberty together was less lonely and scary.

In addition to Emily, I made new friends once my overhand and underhand serves landed me a secure spot on the volleyball team. Teammates became people I called to watch movies and have sleepovers with. Thanks to them, and my friends from youth group, life was awesome in almost every way. There was only one reason it wasn't: I absolutely dreaded going home.

I knew things felt off when Dad moved back home and opened the business, but when Mom and Dad's problems became obvious, I didn't realize at first how deep or far back they went. It took me a while to comprehend what was happening, not only because the fighting was initially secretive, but because we were supposed to be the "perfect" family.

I'd heard of moms and dads not getting along and eventually getting divorced, but that was something that happened to other people, especially people who didn't go to church.

We were the family that prayed before our meals, memorized the Lord's Prayer, and attended harvest parties on Halloween night. I thought we did everything good and right. But as junior high wore on, I realized I'd thought wrong.

When Mom and Dad's late-night "discussions" began, it was clear that something was wrong. Throughout most of my childhood, I'd overheard a quick smooch and softly spoken good nights before my parents drifted off to sleep in their room across the hallway. Yet over time, soft good nights turned into harsh whispers volleyed across the living room. As soon as Andy's and my heads hit our pillows, the defensive conversations, turning into shouting matches, began.

"Why are you fighting?" I'd ask the mornings after arguments, sleepy and nervous for the answer. Andy didn't often ask, making me wonder if I was oversensitive. They didn't realize I was actually setting them up, curious if they'd tell the truth or lie. They'd assumed I'd slept through the disagreement, but little did they know the tension alone kept me awake. I couldn't rest in an unpeaceful house. So I played detective.

Behind my closed door, I'd slide out of bed and press my face against the carpet, my ear in the tiny crack under my door. Unbeknownst to them, I heard why they fought, which I didn't repeat outside the house.

"Oh, they're not fights. We were just having a discussion," Dad usually answered when I'd inquire the next morning.

But I knew better. I'd heard every word.

Although personally rattled, I still wanted to show respect. Although Angel Face, or Punkin Mary as Dad called me, didn't tell the secrets, that didn't mean I wouldn't ask.

"All parents fight," they'd say to justify the arguments.

But I didn't understand. They'd disagreed very little when I was younger, at least in front of me. Did adult-size problems also come with growing up? I couldn't help but wonder as heated chitchats became yelling escapades. When the volume started to really get loud, I had a hunch we'd crossed into abnormal.

School helped mask the tension. Getting lost in an ocean of backpack-wearing junior high students helped moments of home fade away. Giggles and gossip distracted me, as did the cute boys. At school, youth group, or friends' houses, life felt great. But being at home told a different story—a story I couldn't share.

My parents didn't ever need to ask. I'd been trained well enough to know. What happened at home stayed at home, so I didn't talk about their arguing. I stayed quiet when my great grandpa's army cot showed up in the toy room one day so Mom and Dad could take turns sleeping on it. I didn't say "My house is a war zone" when Sunday school teachers asked for prayer requests. When teachers or friends inquired, "What's up with you?" I'd talk about volleyball and walk away.

It felt uncomfortable when people asked about me because at my house, I didn't feel very important.

Somehow, Nick and Leslie from Camp Shamineau picked up on something, although I hadn't said a word. They began to invite me to stay at their house on weekends. It was a nice relief, falling asleep without a tight chest and nervous, aching belly. At their place, I'd laugh at TV shows, eat dinner around a table, pray before bed, and, in general, think.

As I'd snuggle under the covers in their guest bedroom, I'd recognize I felt sad and confused. It didn't add up—how could my family go to church all the time yet live in a constant state of disunity? Frustrated and disappointed at my parents for not acting the way they, or the church, taught me, I felt so thankful for youth camp. Despite my household chaos, I believed God was with me.

I didn't like what was happening in my house, but I came to believe neither did He. And I began to sense God was with me even when I was at home. When I'd hole up in my bedroom, I'd thumb through my Bible looking for verses, and a perfect one would jump out. (The Psalms helped me see other people's families in the Bible weren't so perfect either.) When I prayed, I felt encouraged to find God and look for the good. This became easy in some parts of life, especially fun times with my friend Erin.

We'd become friends through the junior high volleyball team. On the court, she was my favorite setter. She teed up the ball so perfectly, I could easily hit her sets over the net. Our connection on the court led to us becoming good friends. We started hanging out in seventh grade, and once that was over, we saw each other throughout the summers. In eighth grade, we were as close as ever, making the volleyball team once again and getting into club ball. Erin also had only brothers—and I can only assume we acted like sisters. We'd have sleepovers at her house, where we'd wear makeup and take pictures. We'd try out face masks and flip through teen magazines. Toward the end of eighth grade, we'd spend our time dreaming about becoming high schoolers, listening to the radio and watching movies.

"Hey, want to come over and watch *Titanic?* We have the DVD!"

We'd made it to spring break and found ourselves, once again, at Erin's house.

"Yes! Oh my gosh, I love that movie!"

It was an easy answer. My parents would have likely been shocked at my reaction, but deep down, I did love the film. I'd already seen it once—along with almost everyone else in America—but I'd acted uninterested as I walked into and out of the theater. I would have shown more excitement if I weren't going with my family. After the box-office-smashing hype and headlines following the film's release, one unexpected night Mom and Dad took Andy and me to see it at the movie theater. Rarely had we ever gone to a movie as a family. It was so bizarre. To watch a love story, of all types of movies, after my parents had been fighting constantly felt uncomfortable and awkward.

Our city's movie theater in town was dark and musty. The floors were sticky with spilled pop. The red carpet leading into the auditoriums was worn down, and each row was filled with squeaky pull-down seats. It wasn't exactly fun or glamorous. I'd ignored all that when I'd gone to the theater with friends. On those nights it was a magical place. But being forced to watch *Titanic* with my family to my left and a slightly overweight stranger chomping on buttery popcorn and candy to my right, it was miserable. Andy didn't appear happy either. I had a sour attitude, and everyone knew it—I couldn't hide my frown. I kept my head down and my mouth shut. Finally the black screen lit up. It was hard to sit through the show.

As the movie unfolded, the relationship between the two main characters, Jack and Rose, mirrored my own life in eerie ways. One moment they felt happy and hopeful. Their lives were full of dreams. But the next, they were in despair. All their future plans were sinking deep into an icy ocean. I could relate. It was what being a teenager living at my house felt like. One minute, I was excited to grow up and get older. My world was full of hope and wonder. But the next moment, I felt dark, gloomy, and broken down.

I tried not to cry. I didn't want anyone, especially my family, to see how the movie affected me: the sadness, loss, and grief. Although the movie sparked difficult emotions, I still loved the story. The way Jack loved Rose. The way Rose craved adventure and was willing to lose everything to follow her heart. How could I not love it? I was eager to see it again.

I nestled into a corner seat on Erin's couch as she pushed play. Her living room was right next to the kitchen, and the smell of microwave popcorn wafted out. The film's score began piping through the speakers on her big-screen TV, and it made my heart flutter. The scene opened, and there was Jack sneaking his way onto a huge ship, his destiny awaiting him. After a while, the beautiful red-lipped Rose appeared, and they fell in love. It didn't take me long to get into the story, but this time, I let myself ride the waves with them and actually *feel* Rose's temptation to jump after feeling trapped in her picture-perfect life. The hope that she and Jack would get her parents' blessing as they fell in love. As the scenes unfolded, I got caught up in their story, but then I felt a strange flutter race across my stomach.

Shifting my weight on the couch, I tried to ignore it and tune back in to the show.

But a few seconds later, it fluttered again, and I realized what was happening. I had to "go."

Seriously? I'm going to go to the bathroom here? I thought angrily. I was mad at my body for not holding it. I got off the couch and tiptoed into a small bathroom behind us next to the kitchen. I felt a little better that it was just Erin and me at her house, and I prayed none of her family would be home any time soon. I tried to go quickly, yet as I sat on the toilet, I stewed as I studied the wallpaper's detail.

I felt so embarrassed to be pooping at a friend's house. Along with shopping for a bra, starting my period, and performing with little kids at church, this had just made my list of all-time most embarrassing moments.

There was only one reason I wanted to be home,

and this was it—I hated going number two anywhere else. Unfortunately, I had no choice. Fortunately, I went quickly.

As I got up to flush and wash my hands, something caught my eye: a speck of red was floating in the toilet bowl. I didn't typically study my bathroom trips, but I'd happened to glance and see it.

Oh no—this can't be happening. I don't have any pads on me.

Although Erin was a good friend, I rarely talked about my period. Bleeding still made me extremely weary and uncomfortable. My friends at school talked about it freely. They'd even sit in little groups and make nicknames for it like Aunt Flo or On the Rag. But I didn't join them. It was too embarrassing, and I couldn't find the courage to reveal when I went on and off my cycle. Too bashful to ask for help, even at Erin's house, I quickly fixed my problem by substituting a big wad of toilet paper for a maxi pad.

This will have to work until I get home.

I flushed and tiptoed through the kitchen to take my place back on the couch. Although there was still some popcorn in my bowl, my hunger was suddenly gone. I tried to get back into the movie, but my mind raced with anxious thoughts.

Is this toilet paper going to work? What if it leaks? Should I go home now? I don't want to say anything.

The toilet paper was worse than the big, fluffy pad I'd used the first day I'd started. Uncomfortable and distracted, I tried to sit still.

"Hey, I think I'm going to call my mom and head home. I don't feel good," I lied once the credits started scrolling across the screen. Well, technically I didn't feel good—but for other reasons. Normally I would have stayed at Erin's house well into the evening. But with a wad of toilet paper crammed into my underwear, I was ready to go.

Fortunately, we lived close, and Mom picked me up quickly. I didn't say much on the drive home, and I bolted for the bathroom once our car pulled into the driveway. Rushing up two sets of stairs and into my parents' bathroom, I took a deep breath, sat on the toilet, and braced myself.

Huh. That's weird, I thought as I stared down at a wad of white toilet paper.

There was not even one drop of blood. It had been a false alarm. Relieved, I flushed and went to my bedroom. I was exhausted after the anxious afternoon. Breathing deeply, I was glad my body was cooperating—finally. Yet I shouldn't have breathed too deeply that day, for *Titanic* was also trying to tell me something. The tip of an iceberg can be easily underestimated and misleading.

6

Red

*I*T'S GOTTA BE THE RED *licorice.*

I sat in our hallway bathroom and wrinkled my forehead in ignorance and frustration. Another spot of red had shown up unannounced in the toilet. I had thought it a fluke when I first saw the red speck at Erin's house, but a few weeks later, it happened again. And then it began to happen on and off a lot. Throughout the rest of eighth grade, I'd see a red speck—maybe the size of a Frosted Flake—in the toilet once in a while, and even as I started high school and during freshman year, it kept happening. And while the first red specks seemed to float in the toilet water and appear out of nowhere, there was a consistent trend. I noticed the red specks only after I pooped.

Although I was embarrassed to use the restroom in

the first place, it didn't stop me from examining what I flushed. Ever since the first speck of red appeared, I'd developed a habit of looking down.

If anyone walks in on me doing this, I will die, I'd think behind the closed bathroom door. But I was perplexed about what I kept seeing. Eventually, I had other ideas.

Is this even blood? Maybe it's something else.

Desperate for an answer, and for my body to be healthy, I began to come up with other ideas as to what I could be seeing. One day as I sat on the toilet after yet another disappointing sight, I had a brilliant idea. I knew what it was: Twizzlers!

To feed two growing teenagers, my parents shopped at Sam's Club. I played volleyball and Andy played football, and we were hungry all the time. Big boxes of snacks and treats filled our basement each week. Among the bags of chips and cookies sat a jumbo-sized tub of red licorice. It was my favorite snack, and I often snuck downstairs to grab several handfuls each day.

"Slow down on that licorice. It's a lot of candy to be eating."

Mom noticed how much candy I ate, yet while she told me to stop, I couldn't help myself. Not only did I like the licorice so much, but it was difficult to listen to anything Mom said. Her fights with Dad had gotten worse. I'd overheard she didn't love him anymore. They called for help to settle disputes. Why would I stop eating Twizzlers if they couldn't get along without arguing?

Though I hated to admit it, I wondered if Mom was right. Maybe I was eating too much licorice and it was causing the red in my stools. So I decided to try a little experiment to see if I could make my "red problem" go away. I stopped eating licorice altogether. One day I just went cold turkey. I fought the temptation to sneak to the basement for candy. A day or two later, when I felt the urge to go again, I made my way to the toilet and hoped for a success.

> *Maybe I was eating too much licorice and it was causing the red in my stools.*

After doing my business, I did my routine turn around and check, and to my delight, there was no red. Rejoice! Although it was a victory, I celebrated in silence. I didn't want any knocks on the door and questions like, Everything all right in there? Are you okay?

Unfortunately, the victory didn't last long. I didn't go poop every day, so a few days later, when I had to go again, my little red problem was back. A pain of defeat hit immediately. It was both a shock to my chest and a punch to my gut all at once. Not only had my Twizzlers boycott failed, but the red specks were becoming more and more frequent. It became unusual if I didn't see red when I went number two, even if it was just a little. I wasn't sure what to do next, but one thing was certain—I couldn't tell anyone.

Don't cause a fuss—your house doesn't need any more drama.

I talked to myself a lot. I always had. Although I had a brother to play with, I often played alone. I carried a story and constantly heard a narrator in my head. As I got older, I began to recognize the different inner voices. Some were coming from me and how I felt, others were from God, and yet others were from an enemy who didn't like me very much. The voice that got embarrassed about puberty often made convincing arguments about why I needed to hide what went on with my body. I had thought about telling my parents about the red specks, but that meant admitting to looking at my poop—and letting them into my personal life. I wasn't up for either one of those things, so I stayed quiet.

My parents didn't want people knowing about their issues, and I didn't want them knowing about my poop, so I decided to find other ways to fix my body on my own.

What else do I eat that's red?

I wasn't sold on the idea that the red specks meant blood. I liked the idea that they could be appearing because of something else. I made a mental list of red foods—spaghetti sauce, pizza, ketchup, salsa, raspberry popsicles, and strawberries. If the Twizzlers weren't to blame for the red specks, maybe the other red foods were. For the next few weeks, I didn't put anything red into my mouth. (I even avoided cinnamon gum, just to be safe.) I let Andy eat all the bagel bites we cooked for our after-school snack, and I didn't dip my chicken nuggets into ketchup.

I scrutinized every bite, a flashback to my sal-ad-dumping days, making sure no hint of red could be seen. I pushed away the voices telling me "This plan is silly and childish—it's not going to work." I prayed for my no-red-foods diet to fix me and asked God to make the red stop. And for the first week or so, it did. It was a miracle—the red specks were suddenly gone. I'd get even closer to the toilet bowl just to be safe, but from what I could see, the red had gone away. Hallelujah!

But just like my plan with the licorice, my victory was short lived. I wanted to cry when I went to the bathroom one day, looked back, and noticed more red. I refused to let the tears come, although my chest grew sad and heavy. As I flushed it all away, I felt so defeated. The porcelain throne was no place of royalty.

On the outside, I looked perfectly fine and healthy. My freshman year was going well. With my parents' issues aside, I was happy. Classes were relatively easy, volleyball kept me active, and Dad even took me shopping for a homecoming dress—a long, strappy gown—that helped me feel like a real princess.

Although a lot of things were going well for me, on the inside I knew something was wrong. Deep down, I knew I was seeing blood. I wasn't surprised when my food elimination diets failed, just disappointed. But I was already good at putting a smile on my face. I just applied my tricks of hiding my home life to my body. The blood became my little secret for the entire school year, and nobody knew. The more I saw it, the more familiar and comfortable it became.

After a while, an inner voice made a convincing observation. *It's just a little blood. How bad can that be?*

I sat in the darkness behind a red velvet curtain. Warm-up sounds from friends playing tubas and trumpets collided with those of flutes and piccolos as the orchestra indicated it was time for the audience to take their seats. The high school auditorium was filled with parents and friends holding colorful flower bouquets. Dressed in black from head to toe, I took my special seat—a metal stool behind a music stand—and adjusted my headphones to hear the stage crew talking to the booth.

"Okay, show's going to start. Stagehands ready; spotlight in position. Danielle, we're listening for you." I'd rarely held so much power and control.

I was the stage manager of our school's fall musical, and the entire company waited for my cue. My eyes scanned the shadows in the darkness, and I looked for our leads to appear. Smells from crinkly polyester outfits and aerosol hairspray told me the cast and ensemble of our show, *Crazy For You*, was ready.

"Three, two, one, *showtime!*"

The clarinets joined the trombones and drums in a perfect melody. It drowned out the sound of the overhead pulley systems dropping down a western city backdrop. Characters took the stage and began to dazzle the audience—just like we'd practiced in rehearsals. The colorful cast filed into the wings and then danced their way onto the stage.

With the show underway, I sat back and smiled—taking my first exhale of the night.

How did I get here? I could hardly believe it.

My journey into theater had come as a big surprise.

For one, I had refused to act again after my embarrassing church performance. And two, I was only a sophomore running the show. But after taking a freshman theater class, I was introduced to the world of backstage. I tried it during the spring play and found out it really fit me. I became friends with two funny guys named Darren and Daren, and my childhood friend Jordan from the bus to Camp Shamineau acted too. It felt especially nice to join theater after I'd quit sports. Playing the tomboyish athlete was no longer something I could do.

After five years of volleyball and even more years of sports, I stopped playing after my freshman year. I'd kicked off the season with a thigh injury and never quite bounced back. Although I loved the game, each day after school, I felt exhausted. I dreaded staying after school for practice. I just wanted to go home. (Little did I know feeling so tired after school wasn't normal—I mean, who knew about anemia?)

Despite playing in competitive leagues, my skills seemed to get worse. I couldn't jump as high or hit as hard, yet I'd been training and was supposed to be in the best shape of my life. It was slightly embarrassing to go from being a top player in junior high to the B team bench my freshman year. Something was off, but I didn't know what. I hadn't ever connected it to the bleeding.

When our season ended, I felt relieved. I made the decision to quit playing. I looked forward to going home after school so I could lie on the couch and rest. Yet a few months later, when the spring play began, my theater teacher asked me to help with props. Although it required staying after school for rehearsals, it wasn't as exhausting as volleyball. I soon learned why theater groups often call themselves family. I was honored when they trusted me to run the musical a few months later during my sophomore year.

Flutes signaled that the act onstage was about to change, and I cued the lights and stagehands. Dancers dressed as Folly girls wearing blond wigs, bright-pink leotards, and even pinker lipstick soon danced their way into the spotlight. The musical was going perfectly—the audience was laughing, the actors were nailing their lines, and the stage and lighting crews were in sync. As the pulley systems let down a new backdrop and the cast switched out, suddenly I felt a searing stomach pain.

I bent over, careful to not let out any sound. I gripped the top of the music stand, and suddenly, another wave came again. I bent over even farther, curling in my stomach. I'd never felt anything like this.

Did someone just stab me with a knife?

The sharp pains kept coming and traveled all down my legs and throughout my back. Trying to stay silent and not draw any attention to myself, I closed my eyes, gripped the music stand to steady myself as I stood up, and tried to breathe. The pains were so fierce, they took my breath away.

Fortunately, breathing deeply helped, and the pains fizzled out. I sat quietly and alone in the dark corner. Nobody had seen what had just happened. Thank goodness.

What on earth was that?

Once the pain subsided, I rubbed my stomach and sat back on the stool. Flipping through the script's pages,

I caught up with the show. I didn't want to let down any actors if they got stuck and lost their lines. We were in the middle of a performance—what else was I going to do? Not until the actors took a bow and the velvet curtain closed did I deeply, fully exhale. Although my parents were both in the audience, I kept it to myself. My stomach was a little sore, but I felt fine. Plus, I didn't want to miss the cast party.

Yet a few nights later, when sharp pains struck again, fear persuaded me to share. Despite what I wanted to do—and what the inner voice kept telling me—I told somebody.

I took a few cautious steps downstairs to talk to Mom, who was sitting at the computer. I was finally scared enough to break my silence. I'd become used to seeing the red specks—it had been almost two years since I first saw them at Erin's house—but when the sharp pains began, I also started to notice more blood. And it was starting to get darker. There was no questioning it anymore. It was blood, not red foods or dyes. I saw it nearly every time I went poop. I feared using the restroom every few days.

Knowing it likely contained the information, I thought, maybe, our desktop computer could help. I didn't care for computers much, but I was getting desperate. The initial lesson about technology, the one with the funny floppy disk, was cute and all, but a lot had changed since then.

In the midst of many conversations and "discussions,"

Mom uncovered a passion for teaching and returned to college to get certified. Upon her enrollment, we bought our own desktop computer for the house, something way more sophisticated than the typewriter and word processor I'd used for my fourth-grade plays and stories. With an internet-enabled computer at home, we installed a second phone line for dial-up. Andy and I wanted to use it so we could each call a friend at the same time, responding to messages they'd sent us on our pagers. But we understood the line was mostly for Mom's classes and homework. The phone line I wanted to use. But the computer? Not so much.

For starters, the computer took Mom away from me. The screen made me invisible. But more than that, I knew what the internet housed, and I didn't trust it one bit. Early in elementary school, my teacher walked our class to a computer lab that was lined with state-of-the-art technology so we could explore websites. Despite our lesson about how to search online carefully, it didn't stop what happened. I thought I was going to see a picture of the United States president's house when I typed in a URL. But instead of seeing a big white building, I saw nearly-naked girls in swimsuits and lots of stars.

I squirmed in my chair across from a glowing screen of shame. I'd just visited the kind of website my teachers said to avoid. It wasn't on purpose, yet my cheeks couldn't help but flush. Although my teacher reassured me, "You're not in trouble; I know it was an accident," I left the computer lab rattled and mad.

While my classmates grew to love the internet, I had never made amends. Yet I couldn't deny the uncanny parallel growth track between computers and me. Between my time in elementary school and high school, everything about technology also grew up. Computers went from big, expensive devices used at Dad's work to personal desktop computers at home with games like Oregon Trail and Where in the World Is Carmen San Diego? By the time I reached junior high, Andy and I used computers to type homework assignments (for our tech-savvy teachers who required that). By high school, nearly all our friends owned at least one computer, sometimes even a laptop, and we used them for everything—illegally downloading music (oops!), storing photos, playing games, sending emails, and talking through Instant Messenger and chat rooms. Although I didn't like the technology because the shame never fully went away, I didn't want to miss out. So I learned how to type and occasionally logged on.

"It's like the new encyclopedia," one of my high school teachers insisted during a lesson on Internet Explorer and how to put in a URL and use a search bar. I couldn't argue. From what I could tell, the internet did house a lot of answers. One day it hit me.

Maybe the internet can explain my bleeding.

Still uncomfortable with internet searches, I knew Mom would be able to help. So one night after my shower, I snuck down before bed and interrupted her at the computer desk. "If you have time, can you look up something for me? It's not a big deal, but I've been noticing a little blood when I go to the bathroom—and it's only when I go number two."

Mom pivoted away from the screen, looking startled and somewhat confused. I knew she wasn't expecting me to come downstairs in the first place, and certainly not with this request—or news. "Sure. I'll look into it and let you know what I find."

She didn't give much of a reaction and soon turned back to the screen. A few nights later, she called me back downstairs before bed. "Danielle, how much blood are you seeing?"

She was holding printouts in her hand after looking up some information. I took a big gulp and scrambled for an answer, not wanting to reveal the full truth. The last thing I needed was to get chewed out for not telling I saw blood when I pooped sooner.

"Um, just a little bit here and there—not all the time, but sometimes."

It was mostly the truth. I could tell she was pleased by my answer, and I immediately felt relief.

"I found something called 'hemorrhoids,' and they can cause a symptom of 'blood in the stool.'"

Once she said it, I knew immediately. That was it. I had "blood in the stool."

The last thing I needed was to get chewed out for not telling I saw blood when I pooped sooner.

"Hemorrhoids can make you see blood. They're little bumps that can cause bleeding."

Although I didn't have any of the itching and burning that was said to go along with hemorrhoids, everything made total sense. I assumed playing volleyball had given them to me. No wonder I couldn't play very well anymore.

"That's most of the information I found . . . especially for someone your age," she said. She casually mentioned finding a few other causes of blood in the stool, but it could mean something really serious . . . and usually only for people grandma's and grandpa's age.

A jolt went through my body. Serious conditions? I knew I'd severely downplayed the amount of blood. But not wanting to talk any longer, I turned and went back upstairs. I wanted to have hemorrhoids, as awkward as that sounded.

"Thanks again for looking that up!"

Relieved to finally have an answer, I now felt the blood wasn't so concerning. I didn't bring my little red problem up again because we'd discovered what was behind it. For the days and weeks that followed, the red specks continued to appear, but I didn't panic or feel nervous. They were evidence of my hemorrhoids.

Over time, the blood began to change again, which seemed normal to me. It was following its typical pattern—it shifted every few years. At Erin's house, it was a tiny red speck. A few years later, the specks weren't so tiny and bright anymore. The blood turned pretty dark, sometimes even black, and even more was coming. Yet in the midst of it, the blood in the stool wasn't the only thing changing.

Once again, I was going through major changes. Although puberty had come and gone, leaving me a fully grown woman, I was turning sixteen and feeling a new sense of freedom thanks to a driver's license and new-to-me car I called Ruby. Plus, a guy nicknamed Mikey B was taking a lot of my time. With him in my world, I nearly forgot about everything else.

7

Mikey B

THE AUGUST WIND BLEW IN a gentle breeze, making it nice to be outside despite the midwestern Missouri humidity. While Dad mowed, the smell of freshly cut grass wafted through our yard—a nostalgic backdrop to the memory lane I found swirling in as I rummaged through garage storage bins. A tangled volleyball net sparked fond memories of backyard games, and the pink Skip-It reminded me of times I'd felt most confident (I could spin my leg and jump over the incoming ball really fast). Lost in childhood, I paid no attention to the buzzing speakers blaring down the street until a white 1990s Toyota Tercel wheeled into our driveway.

Erin's head popped over the dashboard as she waved. My stomach dropped—*This* must be *him*. In just a few days, freshman classes would begin. Since Erin played in marching band, she'd already been to the high school. Each night she called to dish about band practice, mostly the guys. I was surprised and a little jealous about the senior guys interested in her, although I wasn't surprised. She was gorgeous—big eyes, bouncy hair, and a body that guys called hot. She was often described in ways I'd once dreamed about guys saying about me, dreams I'd let go.

"You would really like Mike, a trombone player. He's a senior, and he wears one of those bracelets that say FROG—Fully Rely on God!"

Knowing faith was important to me, Erin insisted I too would befriend one of the guys. I had my doubts. I didn't want to meet him, but I realized I didn't have a choice as his car drove into our driveway. Not wanting to be rude, I left the Skip-It and walked down to say hello. Erin quickly got out of the car, full of adrenaline. Her dad didn't let her go out with boys much—*this* was new. As we started talking, Mike opened his car door and quietly stepped out. He met us at the hood, and I noticed he was not much taller than me. He had short brown hair, really tan skin, and pretty blue eyes. I liked his white striped Adidas shoes, which made him approachable and friendly. Looking up and down, I searched for any reason to not trust him. His chain wallet made me question him a little, and I became very curious about his silver-balled necklace with an engraved bottle cap. I couldn't read it, but outside of those two things, he did seem safe. He didn't say much and stood around as Erin and I talked.

"We're just driving around. Dad said I've got to be back soon."

Erin was lit up like a Christmas tree, and I couldn't blame her. I still couldn't believe she'd gotten to leave her house with Mike—alone. Although skeptical about his intentions, I couldn't blame Erin for wanting to hang with him. He did seem trustworthy. And she hadn't called it a "date." As far as I knew, they were just friends.

"Bye! See you later!"

Erin returned to the passenger seat, and Mike said, "Goodbye."

Maybe he's not so bad after all, I tried to convince myself as they drove off. Although quiet, he did seem nice.

Yet as school got started and Erin made more friends, she eventually stopped talking about the senior guys. I'd nearly forgotten about Mike until several months later when we ran into each other again.

It didn't take long to learn that in high school, friend groups were everything. The key to surviving. These friend groups seemed to form quickly too. The musicians, athletes, and those who smoked pot all found one another—and fast. Yet as I watched the groups firm up throughout my freshman year, I couldn't quite find my fit.

Most of my good friends were from church, not school. Once Erin joined the band, she hung with other musicians, and I didn't see her as much. I made the volleyball team, but I mostly saw my teammates during practice.

Fortunately, Emily and I always stuck together. One day she wanted me to meet some girls from choir. "Hey, follow me."

I immediately knew when we'd found the group. A

gaggle of students swarmed around one girl's locker like bees on a hive.

How is this freshman so popular already? I wondered as we took our places on the outside. Soon, somebody noticed Emily and started talking to her. I stood there not saying anything until I distantly recognized the familiar face standing next to me.

"Hey, you're Mike, right? I'm Danielle—Erin's friend."

"Oh, yeah. Hey, how's it going?"

"Good! Are you friends with these guys?"

"Sort of. My friend likes one of the girls, so I came with him."

A senior guy about to graduate was hanging around a bunch of freshmen girls? What a loyal friend. Unlike the first time we met in my driveway, we talked until the bell rang.

"Bye. See you later," I said politely, not expecting to see him again.

But to my surprise, I started running into Mike often. He and his friend kept hanging around the group of girls who became Emily's and my friend group. Once he graduated, Mike and his friend still stuck around. They'd come to pool parties, restaurants, and the movies. Typically, once Mike arrived, we'd end up near each other and talk the entire time.

Mike was easy to talk to and a lot of fun. Also, we had a lot in common. I could see why Erin thought we'd hit it off. We were both "good kids" who didn't drink or do drugs. We shared the same beliefs—about God, faith, and Christian music.

We both thought Five Iron Frenzy and Relient K were some of the greatest bands of all time. At first we only saw each other in a group, but eventually, we hung out without them. We'd go to youth group meetings and volunteer for Serve Days. We'd drive into Kansas City's Midtown for concerts and attend Saturday night youth rallies. When I didn't have a date for homecoming my sophomore year, he offered to take me.

"Are you sure you and Mike aren't together?" friends and family pestered us.

"I'm sure . . . besides, he likes somebody else."

They rarely believed me, but it was the truth. We were simply just friends. Our friendship worked because we made it clear: we had zero feelings for each other. Well, that is, until the one night we stargazed as a sort-of-not-quite-who-were-we-kidding couple. I'd be lying if I said *at least I* didn't feel a tiny spark.

It was a crisp fall evening, and a guy from my science class was hosting a Friday night party. His house sat on the outskirts of our suburb and was surrounded by fields and rolled bales of hay. It wasn't tucked into a neighborhood with sidewalks, streetlights, and cul-de-sacs like the rest of ours. Not at all. The cows mooing in the distance made us feel like we'd definitely left what we considered the city. But inside his basement, it was a different story. The scent of sweaty teenagers and the sound of loud music reminded us we'd not ventured too far from home.

Our group of friends was also going to the party, and Mike offered to pick me up. We knew there wouldn't be alcohol, so we decided to go. Drinking parties weren't our thing, and we stayed clear of that scene. But once we made it to the party, it was certainly *dry*, in more than one way. The video games and loud music weren't *quite* entertaining us. Bored, we shot each other a "let's get out of here" look. We met at the back door and slipped outside where the moon and stars lit the sky. The blue midnight darkness took our collective breath away.

"Hey—follow me! I've got an idea."

Mike jogged around the side of the house toward the gravel drive where he'd parked his car. By the time I caught up, he was searching under the passenger seat for something. He found it: a CD. Sliding it into the stereo, he looked back.

"You coming?"

I smiled, yet hesitated. This was a side of Mike only I knew. With one foot on his back bumper, he hoisted his entire body onto the roof. I'd never seen him do something so adventurous, and I knew others hadn't either. Unsure of his plans at first, once I heard the first song playing, I caught on.

He had found DC Talk's *Supernatural* album, one of our favorites that we'd listened to over and over. The album had sparked several conversations about the wonder and beauty of God.

I hiked my foot on his back bumper to join him on the roof. Carefully, I found a seat—not too close to touch but also not *too* far apart. We didn't lie down; that would have crossed a *major* friendship line. But we propped ourselves up with our arms. As we cocked our heads toward the sky, the songs became the evening's score.

Soft sounds from each track floated into the calm night, but thoughts in my mind and butterflies in my stomach told a different story. The scene was incredibly romantic, but Mike was just my friend, and we'd agreed: nothing more! But then things changed.

"You're a godsend, a blessing from above; you've been godsent to me."

The familiar song took on a whole new meaning as I stargazed alongside my best friend. I couldn't resist the new feelings springing up. Mike was my godsend, a very special person whom I cared about so deeply. A man who knew my heart.

Laughter echoing from behind the house broke the moment as our friends left the party. Before any of them made it to the front, we jumped off the roof, got into Mike's car, and slowly drove away.

I hope nobody saw us.

I didn't need to say it aloud to know Mike was thinking it too.

We hadn't done anything wayward or wrong, but I was aware of what it might've looked like. Two friends sitting on top of a car stargazing without anyone else around? I knew people would be skeptical. But if a crowd of skeptics had formed that night, I might have joined them. Were we still just friends? Or had the rooftop sparked something more?

I couldn't deny the chemistry between us. Something seemed to keep drawing us together. It felt a little supernatural to me too. On the ride home, we let the CD repeat. I didn't say a lot; neither did he. For friends who typically talked nonstop, it was eerily silent. I welcomed the darkness of the night; it hid my face and feelings. Although I'd planned to hide them away and never tell, just as I treated so many other things in my life, they eventually spilled out.

At first it was awkward. No other way to put it. Although Mike and I had by now been hanging out for a few years on Saturday afternoons, we decided that on October 28, 2000, we would go on an official date. Neither one of us expected it, partly because we didn't think we'd see each other much once he moved away to school.

After several of his friends from high school enrolled in a private university, Mike decided to try it, too, since he didn't like the other colleges he'd attended. Although it was more than two hours away, I was excited for him. I was also excited for me. I was about to become an upperclassman.

We'd said a hard, final goodbye in a McDonald's parking lot near the highway, which came with an extra-long hug. As we'd been hanging out pretty often for over a year, I was going to miss him. But I didn't realize how much. Neither did he.

Though he wasn't in town anymore, we talked either by phone, using long-distance calling cards, or Instant Messenger, which was free. We wrote each other notes in spiral-bound notebooks every night (we each had one and swapped them on the weekends), and he'd often page me 07734, which when flipped around read "hello." He'd tell me about his classes, the campus, his roommate, and his hilarious new friends. I'd fill him in on school as well, and how I desperately longed to share my faith. I missed him so much, and I knew he missed me too. Eventually, I recognized and shared my feelings. I couldn't hold them back. While daydreaming during class one afternoon, I wrote a note that put them to words and slid it into his jacket as we hugged goodbye one weekend he came home.

> Mikey B, I can't stop thinking about you, times past and times to come. I'm scared inside for what might become of this, although there is nothing to be scared of. As I think about reality, my mind can't help but wander to the past. I look around the corner and think of how it would be to see you there. A new realization comes to me every day about how much I care for you. "Love" is a word with such depths I don't comprehend. I don't know the future or what it holds. I know I love you, but not the depth. The only thing I am sure of is my love for Christ and the relationships He puts me in. He has arranged for you and me to be best friends continually growing together.

Once he read the note, he called. "I feel the same way."

Our friendship was now indeed something more.

"I told you so!" We knew we'd hear it from friends, even as we didn't want to. Several people had insisted we were a couple all along, but we knew the truth. Not until we exchanged notes and feelings did we have a romantic relationship. But once we did, we had to figure out a whole new way of hanging out.

I'd not been on many official dates (neither had Mike), but we decided to pick both a day and location together. The morning of the date, I wasn't sure what to wear. I'd always pictured a first-date outfit as something stylish, cute, and even somewhat girly. The magazines I still occasionally thumbed through, at both grandmas' houses and the teen subscriptions I pulled from our mailbox, were stuffed full of tips. But as I stared into my closet, nothing felt more unnatural than getting dressed up. So I slipped on my favorite jean shorts and a gray Nebraska Huskers T-shirt I'd purchased while visiting Kristi. With my hair in a high ponytail and barely any makeup, I didn't draw any special attention to the reason I was leaving the house with Mike. My parents were on a need-to-know basis, and Mike and my relationship wasn't yet critical information.

"Later; leaving with Mike," I hollered into the house while walking outside, just as I had so many other times. But on this afternoon, Mike opened the passenger-side car door for me before driving to Kansas City's Country Club Plaza.

I'd lived in Kansas City my whole life, and I'd been to the Plaza dozens of times. At first I'd ridden in a stroller and taken pictures next to artsy penguins. I'd walked around at Christmas to see the lights. But not until I arrived on a fall day had I ever noticed its romanticism. The curves of the Spanish-style buildings, the allure of

fancy shops and restaurants, the beauty of the fountains—it was like a whole new place. Pointing out ornate
statuary, we strolled around other couples and families.
When my stomach grumbled, we realized it was the late
afternoon. We were both hungry.

"Where do you want to go? I'll take you anywhere!"
Mike offered.

But knowing his budget looked a lot like mine,
closer to zero than a hundred, we chose McDonald's so
we could each eat two cheeseburgers and fries for less
than ten dollars. The company alone was satisfying; we
didn't need to eat anywhere fancy. I loved that we could
still be us (and that the Plaza hosted a fast food option).
After lunch, we strolled more and took in why Kansas
City's called City of Fountains. A fall wind kept blow-
ing through town and scattering colorful leaves that had
fallen from wise trees. The scene was stunning, framed
forever in my memory. It was a beautiful day.

Is this more than just friends? I'd catch myself thinking
as we wove in and out of crowds filling the sidewalks. It
felt like so many other times we'd hung out, and our conversations hadn't changed. But as we walked, our bodies
kept inching closer, and at one point, our fingers gently
touched. A few seconds later, his hand reached out for
mine. And in that split second, it became official—we
were *together.*

10-29-00
Dear Danielle (My Diva),
I cannot tell you how many times I've read that
note you wrote me that I keep in my wallet. I got

chills reading it just a few minutes ago. You know, the chills you get when you know God is right there with you. The best feeling in the world. I want you to know that I think the exact same things too. I can't stop thinking about you and times to come. But aren't we always thinking the exact same thing? Thank you for such an awesome weekend. Thank you for being the way you are. The weekend is definitely one of my tops, of all time. Every time I pray, I thank God for you.
—Mikey

I'd be lying if I said it didn't feel odd, suddenly dating my best friend. Our notes to each other had gone from updates between friends to all-out love letters.

As quirky and uncomfortable as being a couple felt at first, especially during our first kiss, it also felt very right. Outside of Emily, Mike was my closest friend. We had already lived through a lot of life. He'd supported me through a couple of boyfriends and breakups, and he prayed for my relationships at school. When the arguing at home got bad, I confided in him. The day he officially became my boyfriend, he practically knew everything about me already . . . well, *al*most everything.

> *I'd be lying if I said it didn't feel odd, suddenly dating my best friend.*

I'd never mentioned my little

bathroom problem. I wasn't comfortable talking to anyone, including Mike, about those details. But when things got really scary as the searing pain returned and frightening amounts of blood followed, I had to say something. I couldn't tell him exactly what it was, so it started out as an unspoken prayer request. But before I knew it, the words flowed from my mouth into the phone's receiver one night.

"I think I need to see a doctor."

10-31-00
Dear Danielle,
As you were about to get offline, you said something to me that no one ever has before. "You are incredible." That is like something someone/everyone waits their whole life to hear (which is a sad thing). But no one has ever said that to me. I had to catch my breath. I was just like, "Wow! Thank you, Lord." I don't know how to respond except that if I am incredible, then you are incredible. Yes, you are. God is doing amazing things. I can't imagine what's to come. You have an unspoken prayer request—I will fall asleep praying for you about it tonight. My dearest Danielle, thank you for being the best, best (x infinity) friend ever. I love you soooooooooo much!
—Michael

8

Busted

WHILE I MIGHT HAVE LOOKED like a fully grown, mature woman to those who didn't know me, at seventeen I still wasn't quite there. Puberty's changes had all arrived—and stayed—but I wasn't mature about *everything*. I still hated to poop anywhere but home, and even there, I dreaded the toilet. I also didn't openly discuss female things. As they both involved bleeding, periods and poop were off limits.

But one night, I couldn't help but bring it up.

The unspoken prayer request to Mike was this: earlier that day, I was sitting at the computer after school chatting with him on Instant Messenger when I let myself pass gas. Andy was with a friend, and both Mom and Dad were still at work. Since Mike was online, he couldn't smell it.

As soon as I let it go, something happened.

"I'll be right back," I typed just before racing up the stairs to the toilet. I sat down to see that I hadn't passed gas, as I'd suspected. To my surprise, there was a large amount of blood.

Oh my gosh. What in the world?

It was worse than getting my period, not only because it was more blood than I'd ever seen, but I didn't understand how or why it was happening. I didn't recall hemorrhoids doing this.

I quickly changed and started the washer to clean my dirty clothes. Once I got back downstairs, I double-checked that I hadn't stained the computer chair and returned to my conversation with Mike.

"Okay, I'm sorry about that. I'm back!"

My fingers were shaking as I tried to type, but eventually my nerves calmed down. I didn't mention it to Mom or Dad later that night, and certainly not Andy. But from that point forward, I was living with terror. Later that night, while on the phone, I realized I had to tell Mike *something.*

I knew he'd pray for me, but honestly, I didn't expect him to remember or care so much. For years, my bathroom issues hadn't been a big deal. When Mom and I discussed them, they didn't seem alarming. But that wasn't the case with Mike.

"Did you call the doctor yet?" He wouldn't stop his asking, both over the phone and on the weekends when he came home.

"No."

It was my constant reply that didn't prevent him from pestering. For over two months, he persisted. One afternoon over his Christmas break, Mom happened to over-hear him while we were hanging out at my house. She inferred what he was talking about (although he person-ally had no clue).

"You're still having those issues?"

Like a deer in the headlights, I froze.

"Yes" is what I actually said. What I wanted to say was quite different: *The tension at home is so thick, these holidays when you and dad barely tolerate each other are mis-erable. I'm just trying to stay out of the way. It's not a big deal—I'm not a big deal. Plus, it's just a hemorrhoid!*

Yet I didn't say that. I just confirmed I was still bleed-ing. Soon after, I regretted saying anything, to anyone, at all.

I couldn't lie, even to myself. The bleeding was get-ting worse. The sharp pains were back too. Except unlike the pains that came during the high school musical, the new pains spread throughout my stomach. They didn't just punch me in the gut once, they lasted all day and all night. I didn't recognize how bad they were at first. I assumed my upset stomach was due to holiday stress and eating lots of bad foods.

For Christmas, we packed up our family sedan, just like always, and drove to a grandparent's house. Although now teenagers, Andy and I still drew lines in the back-seat cushions marking where each of us could and could not cross. Neither one of us wanted to leave home, partly because of our friends, and also because our parents kept fighting. Caged in the backseat for a drive across Missouri, I knew the expectation—it mirrored church. Play along and appear to be a loving family, ignoring the reality Mom and Dad hardly, calmly, spoke. In truth, it had been years since things felt happy. My stomach knotted up just thinking about it. Yet it was similar to the knot I felt after dinner.

Ignoring the "healthy tips" the magazines offered, I loaded up on rich foods and holiday cookies. Grandma Rose Mary's delicious fried chicken, mashed potatoes, rolls, and ramen noodle salad was homestyle cooking at its finest, and mouth-watering good. I'd filled up after our four-hour drive to her farm, yet once I left the table, I regretted eating so much. I couldn't get comfortable while sitting in the recliner, and my chest felt like it was on fire from heartburn. My already-knotted stomach felt even tighter. Once everyone went to bed, I told Mom I wanted to sleep on the couch.

Not only was it closer to the bathroom, but it allowed me to move without waking anyone up. As the house went quiet and dark, I covered up with a colorful homemade afghan and tried to sleep. Yet as the hands on the spinning gold clock kept inching closer and closer to Christmas morning, I tossed and turned in pain.

When the clock chimed at midnight, Santa didn't appear, but I was certain a little man trapped inside my stomach did. It felt like somebody was living inside me and trying to cut their way out. It hurt so badly, the pain took my breath away.

Somehow, finally, it subsided during the early morning hours. The noise of our family greetings, "Merry

Christmas!" and the wafts of brewing coffee got me to sit up and not hog the couch. I tried not to move.

"How did you sleep?" Mom asked, surprised to see my weary face.

I couldn't hide it and eventually broke down and told her. "I'm having really bad stomach pains," I said, pointing to my gut. "It's excruciating."

When the clock chimed at midnight, Santa didn't appear, but I was certain a little man trapped inside my stomach did.

We searched Grandma's medicine cabinet and found an over-the-counter antacid. I drank a capful, hopeful it would help. As the hours wore on and the living room floor became littered with crinkled wrapping paper and new gifts, the little man, fortunately, went away. But days later, once we had made it back home, he came again. Mom bought me more antacid drink, and I started drinking it daily, hoping, praying it would help. I needed a quick cure, not only for my stomach pains, but for my broken heart.

1-21-00

Dear Danielle,

It was a rough month for "us," but I do think it was a good growing experience. I'm sorry, I hate that I've done this; I actually "like" you more when we're apart. I can only see the inside of you when you're away. If I was blind, I'd marry you. I hate that I put the blind thing in. I hate it. What's wrong with me? "I despise my own behavior." Things got off with us. That'll be okay though. In the words of Rob Thomas, we've "got to get back to good." I'm sorry for what's happened and is going on. I don't know what I'd do without you, and I don't want God to show me. You're the only person who will put up with me; you even try to figure me out. God bless you. Pray for me, and I will pray for you. I know God is going to take care of us.

—Michael

Sometimes you just can't hide it.

"Where have you been?"

Dad's eyes were angry, something I wasn't used to seeing when he looked at me. I fumbled for the words, hopeful I wouldn't be asked for the whole story. I wasn't yet ready to tell them about Mike.

"Scott's house. I went over there after school."

Scott was another good friend from church youth group who was two years older than me and also home from college for Christmas break. Throughout high school, we hung out a lot. I usually felt more comfortable hanging out with guys versus girls. There was less drama and no expectation on acting feminine. Whether in his basement playing on his drum set or in his bedroom listening to music, Scott's house was a fun place. As fate would have it, Scott and Mike were enrolled at the same university and even assigned rooms in the same dorm hallway. Living just a few doors down from each other, I missed them both but was thrilled when my two closest guy friends started hanging out. They spent a lot of time together at school, and Scott cheered us on as Mike and I became an official couple.

But then came something I didn't expect over Christmas break. I couldn't believe the words coming out of my mouth. "Mike and I broke up—we're just friends again."

In the midst of a few disagreements, Mike and I decided the long distance that had once pulled us together was not going to hold in person. Truth be told, we'd been friends for so long because we weren't really attracted to each other. I wasn't blond and athletic like the hot girls Mike swooned over. In all fairness, he wasn't tall, dark haired, and tan like some of my previous boyfriends. Despite wanting to be faith-filled teens living for God, we were still . . . well, human. Our conversations were hard, like someone was ripping my heart out. Although we said and wrote "I love you," I had to accept our love was just between friends.

Scott was silly, and he always made me laugh, so I thought a few hours at his house would help cheer me up.

Thanks to love, my junior year had been going blissfully wonderful, but now, just days into the second semester, everything tanked.

My parents didn't typically ask where I went, and I'd not given them reasons to mistrust me, so I went straight to Scott's after school. As I suspected, time with him helped. Noticing the setting sun, I grabbed my backpack and left for home.

Steering into the driveway, I noticed Dad's car and

instantly knew something was wrong. As I opened the door from the garage, I braced myself and listened for another shouting match. It was the only explanation I could think of for why both Mom and Dad were home already, and so early. It wasn't even five o'clock yet. Yet the house was quiet as I walked up the stairs. Once I made my way into the kitchen, I saw Dad with arms crossed and a red face. I was waiting for it.

"Our marriage is over—we're done."

But instead, I heard, "We've been waiting for you—get in the car NOW."

Shocked and stunned, I couldn't fathom how and why *I* was suddenly the problem. I guess I could have called from Scott's house, and I hadn't checked my pager. But still, why was Dad home so early? Where were we going? Where was Andy? My questions didn't get answered until we merged onto the highway.

"We're going to a gastroenterologist, but the office closes soon. They're going to try to stay open for us if we can get there."

A gastro-what? In about two seconds, I realized my little secret had made its way to Dad. Busted. I eventually learned the full story. Once Mom and Dad called my primary care physician's office and explained my symptoms, the nurse insisted I see a gastroenterologist, a GI doctor who treated gut stuff, right away. I couldn't believe the little bleeding problem I'd kept secret for years was suddenly so public.

"Danielle, they need to run a few tests today, and we want you to be prepared," Mom said in an unusually gentle way.

The highway had calmed Dad, much to my relief. I hated him being mad at me. I was so confused and felt caught in a tornado. Although one year away from age eighteen, legal adulthood, I felt like a little kid. Being clueless about doctors and checkups didn't help.

"They might need to do a rectal exam to see where the blood is coming from," Mom added.

A rectal exam?

I didn't react and kept staring out the side of the window. Dad's anger had subsided, but mine was starting.

Frustrated that it was my body, not theirs, I had no choice in what was happening. Rectal? It was such a horrible thought—mortifying. I couldn't fathom it. Surely this wasn't my life.

First, I was in a car, alone with my parents, who couldn't get along. Next, they knew my secret: I saw blood when I went poop. Finally, they were rushing me to a doctor who wanted to examine . . . my butt? I curled up into a little seat-belted ball in the backseat. I didn't know what else to do other than pray. Nothing I could say would change the immediate plan as Dad sped and took sharp right turns.

God, help this nightmare be over soon.

Frustrated that it was my body, not theirs, I had no choice in what was happening. Rectal? It was such a horrible thought—mortifying. I couldn't fathom it. Surely this wasn't my life.

Instant regret fell heavily into my lap and made its home in my chest.

I should have never told Mike about this. I feel fine. I'm not sick.

By the time we arrived at the doctor's office, I'd decided to never tell anyone anything ever again—boyfriend or not. My body was my business, and nobody else's. I didn't need people knowing about or looking at it. But I soon learned this wasn't an option when it came to filling out medical forms and seeing a doctor. As we sat in the lobby and waited our turn, I held a clipboard asking me extremely personal questions such as the date of my last period and what I saw when I went poop. Game over. There was no other way out than forward.

Irony hit as I looked around and realized I was playing Andy's role. He was the one who'd been in the hospital for surgeries and ER visits, not me. Thanks to Andy, Mom and Dad looked like pros. Parking, finding the building, checking in, and getting admitted—it was all new to me but not to them. They knew to sit in the brown, bland waiting room chairs and fill out the worksheets while we waited.

They also knew to stand up and follow the nurse sporting comfortable scrubs when she called my name. "Danielle Ripley?"

Dang it, they really are rushing me in, I said to myself as we stood up and passed other, gray-haired patients who'd been waiting much longer than me.

"Let's get your height and weight."

Dang it again. I hoped for good news as I stepped onto the scale, yet I didn't expect to see it. I'd steadily gained weight over the years, although I kept working out and jogging around the neighborhood. I couldn't seem to shed the extra pounds and sighed in frustration when the scale wasn't 125 like I wanted. After writing down my measurements, the nurse led us into a small room and invited me to take a seat on the tall table covered in crinkly white paper—the kind I drew on at Italian restaurants with crayons. But instead of offering me crayons, she asked me to open up and say *Ahhh*.

"I'm getting your vital signs. The doctor will be in to see you shortly."

Before she left the room, she also wrapped a dark-blue cuff around my arm that squeezed it super tightly—like the machines at the pharmacy—and stuck her cold fingers on my wrist to get my pulse.

How is this happening? I still couldn't believe it.

Knock, knock.

I soon heard two gentle raps against the closed wooden door. In walked a dark-haired, slightly balding man who wore a white coat with "Dr. Marc Taormina" embroidered over the breast pocket. Quickly, he introduced himself and discussed the purpose of the appointment. Although I disliked being in his office, I instantly liked him, even if I didn't care for his particular field of medicine. He talked mostly to my parents, yet occasionally looked to me. They couldn't answer *all* his questions.

"What are you seeing? How much blood? How often?"

They were details that I'd not told a soul, things I hadn't dared to write down or pray about. But lying and hiding had gotten me into his office, and I realized it wouldn't get me out.

Fortunately, Dr. Taormina was patient and seemed

to sense my discomfort. He spoke slowly, kept calm, and didn't react to anything I said, even if the details about seeing so much blood in the stool were alarming. Just as I thought our visit was over (it wasn't so bad), the worst part began.

"I need to do a rectal exam."

Never would I have admitted it, but I was thankful my parents had warned me. The room cleared out so I could get ready alone. I repeated the directions to myself.

Get undressed from the waist down. He needs to examine my bottom. We need to do a test that will tell them if there's blood in my stool.

I shook my head.

That's so silly. They want to test for this? Oh Doctor, you don't need to do this—I can tell you with 100 percent certainty there's blood.

But unfortunately, I had no choice—and neither did he. If we were going to find out why I'd been bleeding, this was a nonnegotiable step one. I changed and sat back on the crinkly paper with a white, scratchy blanket wrapped around my waist. I was thankful when I got to keep my shirt and bra on, my socks too.

Knock, knock.

Dr. Taormina and his nurse were back, and the second they walked in, my heart began to pound. My parents were outside in the hallway waiting, which made it feel even more serious and scary.

"Can you lie on your left side for me?"

The rule-following kid kicked into gear, and I robotically followed his directions. The paper wrinkled as I rolled, and I felt a brush of cold air against my bottom. I was exposed; there was no turning back. I wanted to melt into a mortified puddle. Nobody had seen that area since I'd turned thirteen months old and potty trained myself. Not my parents. Certainly not Andy. Nor Mike.

I took a deep breath and swallowed, and soon I felt someone's hand rest on my hip. I wasn't sure if it was to provide me comfort or to keep me still for what came next. Plastic rubber gloves snapped onto someone's hands, and then I felt pressure and something very cold. Every muscle tensed up despite the encouragement to "breathe and relax." I wasn't exactly sure what kind of tool or testing strip was inserted into my behind, nor did I have the courage to look back or ask. I kept my eyes straight ahead, staring at a white wall and wiggling my toes until it was over. I couldn't help that my body was shaking. Fortunately, the test went fast, and the nurse walked over to comfort me.

"Honey, you can get dressed."

As the room filled back up, nobody made eye contact. Assuming they understood my humiliation, I was not asked how I felt or why I was shaking. Everyone did seem to pity me, and I didn't blame them.

A final set of knocks meant the doctor was back.

"The result is positive for blood."

No duh—I could have told you that was what I wanted to say. I didn't mention I'd been seeing the blood for years, starting as early as eighth grade. Instead I nodded my head like I understood.

He continued, with a concerned look on his face. "I need to do a colonoscopy—and quickly."

9

Scoped

I WAS TOTALLY LYING.

"Why aren't you eating anything?" My friends slid their lunch trays on our round wooden table and noticed I didn't have a tray.

"I'm not very hungry today."

But the truth was, I was starving. Sitting in the high school cafeteria was near torture. The smells of hamburgers and fries, as well as hot, fresh chocolate chip cookies, kept tempting me to eat. But the instructions I'd received, both at the doctor's office and at home earlier that morning before I'd left for school, were clear.

"You must fast all day on Friday."

I'd never fasted, and after only a few hours of it, I didn't ever want to fast again. I didn't know why Mom and Dad voluntarily did it with our church. At the time, I didn't think much about it other than knowing it meant Andy and I would get a special treat. While Mom and

Dad sipped juice all day, Andy and I got special micro-wavable TV dinners. The candy bar dessert (which you removed before zapping) was my favorite.

"Are you sure you're not hungry?"

My friends could tell something was off with me, and they were right, but I wouldn't tell them. My week had already been difficult enough. I didn't need my friends knowing I'd seen a GI and was going to get a colonos-copy the next day. Plus, I hadn't loved hearing the nurse describe the procedure in the GI's office before we left: "a lighted tube with a camera on it" put into my rear so the doctor could take a good look.

Eww and gross. I decided to keep it to myself. Between needing a colonoscopy and not getting to eat all day, my life was going from hard to worse.

While my friends chowed down on their lunches, I sat quietly and stared at the clock. The noise from the cafeteria was especially loud, not only because it was Fri-day, but because the popular kids were across the room. Something about slipping on a letter jacket and sitting at their tables gave both guys and girls permission to laugh, holler, and yell extra loudly. On some days, I looked over and secretly longed to be invited to sit at their table. On other days, I couldn't care less. And on the Friday before my colonoscopy, hours into my fast with even more hours to go, I wanted nothing but to go home.

Friday nights were always one of my favorites grow-ing up. In the years before Mom and Dad's problems began, Fridays brought many of my fondest memories. Most weeks, we'd cook frozen pizzas in the oven and eat off paper plates in the living room. Anything that broke our normal routine felt fun and special. We'd huddle around the TV to watch several hours of the ABC network. We all loved the shows on TGIF—the theme songs got me standing up and dancing each week.

Family Matters usually kicked off the evening—it was one of our favorite shows, thanks to Jaleel White playing Steve Urkel.

"Did I do thaaaaaat?" didn't only make Andy and me laugh, but Dad roared the loudest.

Boy Meets World came after and made me yearn for a best friend like Shawn and a romance like Topanga and Cory's. (Part of why Mike and I hit it off was that he adored the show too and, come to find out, prayed for a best-friend-turned-soulmate like Topanga.)

Many other Friday night shows of my childhood, especially *Step by Step* and *Sister, Sister*, fueled my craving for a teenage life. The cool clothes, updated bedrooms, and freedoms teens apparently had looked so amazing. It wasn't exactly the type of freedom I found myself enjoying the night before my colonoscopy.

Because I was old enough to stay home by myself, I'd asked my family to leave the house during my bowel prep. I hadn't shared many preferences or opinions up until this point, mostly because I didn't think my voice or opinions mattered. I'd not chosen to visit the GI doctor, nor did I have a choice regarding the rectal exam. The colonoscopy was mandatory, as was fasting the day prior to it. Like a test at school, there was no questioning it. But when prep night came—like a total gastro cleanout—I did take back some control and demanded I be left alone.

Not only did I want to avoid smelling my family's dinner, I really didn't want an audience as I ran to the bathroom all night. I didn't want to hear jokes or to be cheered up. I wanted everyone out of my sight. They didn't argue, and to my surprise, they made a plan for all of them to go to dinner.

"Okay, but I'm going to watch you take the first dose before I leave."

Although I'd never been rebellious, it was as though Mom had read my mind. I debated not drinking the prep liquid once they left (neglecting to think through what would happen if I didn't take it).

In the brief instructions given by the nurse at the GI's office, she'd said to buy clear liquids and hinted that I might not like the taste. I stood over the kitchen sink and grabbed a plastic cup to get started. I took a small bottle of clear, bubbly liquid and mixed it in the cup with Sprite, hoping my favorite soft drink would mask any bad taste. It fizzed as the liquids mixed together. I gripped the cup tightly and took a big sip. And then I nearly spit it all out over the window above the sink.

But when prep night came—like a total gastro cleanout—I did take back some control and demanded I be left alone.

"*Mmummhokhm.*" I was shaking my head rapidly, my

face twisting in agony as I tried to signal and say, "I'm not going to get this down my throat." My head bobbled in horror, my stomach started to flip, and my throat tightened up. My body did not want the awful liquid to come in.

"Come on, you can do it. Drink it down." Mom's feeble attempt to coach me wasn't working. She had never tried to do this—nobody in the family had ever had a colonoscopy. Poison—or ocean water—I became convinced that was what went into my mouth. In nothing short of a miracle, I breathed through my nose and somehow got it down. It burned my taste buds and made me want to vomit. I'd never tasted anything so horrible—not even the night I was forced to eat sauerkraut and subsequently threw it up in the sink.

"I'm sorry, Angel Face."

Angel Face? Mom really did feel bad. As she attempted to offer more encouragement, I braced the sides of the sink and looked down. I couldn't do it—there was no way I could take another drink. She rubbed my back for a few minutes before reminding me I had to complete it.

I'm not sure how, but I eventually grabbed a straw and added ice cubes to force down the rest of the prep drink. Alternating between big gulps and small gulps, I also mentally recited Bible verses and worship songs. By the time the slurps came from the bottom of the cup, I wasn't sure if I needed to lie down on the couch or continue to stand hunched over the sink. My bloated gut filled, and I stood still. A few minutes later, it settled.

"I promise I'll finish the remaining prep if you go."

Mom grabbed her purse and called for Dad and Andy, who'd stayed far away from the kitchen. I could tell she was doubtful, but she knew I wasn't kidding. I wasn't exactly in a joking mood.

They finally left, and I curled up into a ball on the living room couch. It was hard to hold back the tears that welled inside. I felt sorry for myself. I felt as if I were being punished, but for a crime I didn't do.

Why am I bleeding? It's not my fault. Why did I need to visit the doctor? And why did I need that rectal exam? It was so awful. I've been a good kid all my life, a Christian who likes church and reads the Bible. I love God. Why am I going through this?

My pity party continued.

Sure, I didn't tell anyone about the blood, and I downplayed what was going on. Maybe I stretched the truth, but who can blame me with everything else that goes on at my house?

Suddenly, a faint ripple ran across my abdomen—like a bubble-growl that morphed out of nowhere. Another came. And another. I rushed to the bathroom for the first of several trips, which crashed my pity party. And several more.

"How did your prep go?"

Surrounded by beeping machines pumping IV fluids into my arm, I realized Mom was right. Warm blankets at the hospital are wonderful. I was tired and drained, and I felt like a walking raisin, only I was lying in a medical bed with guardrails. My fingers were even crinkly, I was so dehydrated. After twelve hours of constantly rushing to the bathroom, I was shriveled up and ready to feel normal again.

"Good," I said in a hurried one-word reply that seemed to appease the nurse. I wasn't up for chit-chat, and she could tell.

Something was terribly wrong with me. What could it be? I had no idea. But I couldn't deny the problem anymore.

Truth was, I didn't want to share the details of my evening. I almost didn't believe them myself.

I'd seen a lot of blood whooshing out of me—way more than I expected. By the time I finally started "running clear" hours into prep night, meaning what came out of me looked like water, my hands were shaking. Mike's surprise visit (which I kept short and made him stay at the front door) helped. But it didn't take away the fear.

Something was terribly wrong with me. What could it be? I had no idea. But I couldn't deny the problem anymore. As we checked into the hospital, I'd become very compliant.

Like the doctor's office, the hospital was new to me. Wheels from other patients' beds rolled down the hallways, and the rubber soles on the nurses' shoes squeaked when they approached my bed. The curtains, charts, computers, and gowns. The rubbing alcohol pads, pokes, and small sticks. I'd just stepped into a whole new world. Once again, this was Andy's world—not mine. It didn't feel real. Luckily for him, he was at home asleep while I was the one in the hospital this time (getting a tube stuffed up my rear). My, how the tables had turned.

The promise of my red problem going away helped me deal with everything going on around me. The staff working in the outpatient clinic had been quiet, and in my view, slightly awkward. But I guess it made sense. Seventeen-year-olds didn't typically roll in to get colonoscopies early on Saturday mornings. Most of the staff scrambled for the words to say when they tried talking to me, all except for Nurse Lori.

"Hi, Danielle! I'm Lori. You're friends with my daughter. I'll be with you during your colonoscopy today. I'll be here the whole time."

Like a bright ray of sunshine, Lori appeared just after I was wheeled back into the procedure room. Her daughter was a friend who hung out with Mike's and my group. Instant relief washed over me as Lori gently brushed the back of my hand; her motherly smile reassured me everything was going to be okay.

I looked around the room to figure out where I'd been taken. A small TV monitor was to my right, along with a long, black snakelike tube. I assumed this was the tube with a camera at the end that the nurses had told me about—the one I dared not mention to my scarfing lunchroom friends. I knew where it had been and where it was going next. Gross.

A metal tray was situated next to the tube with an oversized paper napkin on it. A nurse walked over to the tray and casually squirted a big pile of clear jelly onto the napkin. It sounded like a big fart, and I barely stifled a laugh—for the first time in several days, something was funny.

A lot of people kept moving in and out of the room, all wearing scrubs and smiling. I had no idea who they were or what their jobs were, but with Lori standing next to me, I didn't really care. Dr. Taormina entered the room along with an anesthesiologist, who then explained what was happening as a clear liquid flowed through the tiny tube connected to my vein.

"You might start to feel a little fuzzy and dizzy. That's normal."

If so, I thought, *that's about the only thing that's normal around here.*

The room started to spin, and a dark tunnel appeared in my mind's eye. The light at the end was growing fainter and farther away. In what felt like only a minute later, I opened my eyes to very bright lights in a different room, pats on the arm, and new beeping sounds. I struggled to stay awake. Mom and Dad's faces became clear. The colonoscopy was over.

Once I could keep my eyes open, the nurses disconnected my tubes. I still felt super groggy from the medicine, and my stomach was as bloated as a balloon. My parents kept acting a little weird, but that wasn't unusual. I was used to seeing them act strange around each other. I figured sitting in a waiting room together hadn't gone so well. Yet I didn't sense they'd been fighting. On the contrary, they acted close and were getting along. Something was off.

"You doing okay? Can I get you anything?"

Once I'd woken up, they were both very attentive.

Dad couldn't stop rubbing my arm. Mom stayed near my head and fed me ice chips. They both teased me about mentioning Nurse Lori multiple times—something the nurses reassured us was normal.

"You can go ahead and get dressed," the nurse directed.

Finally, I thought. *I'm starving.*

While I was focused on drinking my Sprite and staying awake, Dr. Taormina stopped by to hand my parents a folder. I assumed he'd spoken to them during one of the times I fell back asleep. Dad took the folder as Mom helped me get off the bed and stand to get dressed. A whole crew of nurses walked to the front doors, and I eventually made it to the car.

"Did he find what caused the bleeding?"

Focused on leaving the hospital, getting dressed, and eating again, I hadn't thought to ask for the results until we were almost home. I assumed no news was good news. (Wrong!)

Mom and Dad looked back and forth at each other, and then straight ahead.

"Sort of. The doctor found something, and he is sending it off for testing. We won't know anything for a few days," Dad replied.

The answer had been given so quickly and nonchalantly I didn't think anything about it. It didn't seem serious, whatever it was, so I decided not to worry.

Finally. I won't see blood anymore, I thought as we drove home in an unusually quiet car. Thing is, I hadn't fully understood that the colonoscopy itself hadn't fixed anything—it just showed us what was there, deep inside.

10

Cancer

"**I**S IT TRUE? YOU HAVE cancer?"
The question caught me off guard, as did those that followed.

"Danielle, did you have a procedure yesterday? We heard about it, and we heard it could be cancer."

The whispers from my Sunday school teachers in the hallway outside the church's youth room were low, yet serious. Although I'd spent almost all of Saturday sleeping on the couch once I got home from my colonoscopy and gave Mike the update, by Sunday morning, I felt normal again and went to church with my family.

While we didn't do many things together anymore, we hardly missed church. I was expecting to slip into youth group without anyone knowing what I'd done the day before, threatening Andy not to tell. But apparently some phone calls had been made while I was riding out my Saturday fog.

Cancer? The thought never crossed my mind. My parents didn't mention anything about cancer to me—that would have been major—and serious! I quickly eased their fears. "No, it's not cancer. I had a colonoscopy yesterday, and the doctor found something. He's sending it on for more tests. But I don't think it's cancer."

They looked relieved, and I was too once I saw my friends and rushed off to sit next to them. As the worship band started to play, I couldn't help but wonder why I'd just been asked if I had *cancer*. That word had *never* come up.

Surely Mom and Dad would have mentioned cancer . . . I don't have cancer—right?

The band began playing, and a room of fellow teenagers standing up to sing and clap took my focus away from the worry. Every second of youth group was enjoyable to me; I couldn't really explain why. A lot of my friends—and my brother, truth be told—were bored with church after growing up in it. But the love for God I'd found at Camp Shamineau never went away. Despite the chaos at home, my faith in God stayed strong. I knew God was going to take care of me. It was something Mike, despite being my ex-boyfriend now, reminded me of constantly. Although we'd returned to just friends, we still talked every night and swapped journals on the weekends. He was the only person I confided in about the colonoscopy, and he promised to pray.

"Go to your classes!"

The worship set ended, and a river of students flowed into guys' and girls' Sunday school classrooms. Nervous for my leaders to comment during class, I felt relief when they didn't say a peep about my scan or *cancer threat*. Once classes dismissed, Andy and I found Mom and Dad upstairs, and we shuffled through the crowded hallways toward a huge auditorium lined with comfortable stadium-style seats. I didn't love "big church" as much as youth group, and I missed the smaller pew-lined churches from my childhood days. Unlike the megachurch we'd started attending, the people in the smaller churches knew my name. But there was no denying it: the cushioned seats were really comfortable.

A robed choir filed onstage and service began. We sang a couple of songs before sitting down for the sermon. My body was weak, dehydrated, and tired from the colonoscopy. I couldn't focus. My mind kept wandering back to the harrowing question I was unsuccessfully avoiding.

Do I have cancer?

Mom's hand wrapped around my arm brought my attention back to the auditorium. I'd zoned out for the entire thing.

As the final songs began and the church issued its altar call, I got another funny feeling. "Danielle, let's go up to the front and pray."

I still disliked altar calls. They'd never grown on me, although they'd come to include receiving prayer for any life hardship in addition to praying for salvation. Dad's hand was on my back as he whispered in my ear. Something was very weird and not right. They knew I was shy and didn't like being in front of people. I wanted to freeze, to sit down to protest. But once again, I didn't *really* have a choice. Mom and Dad were on the same page, which was also strange. I could do nothing but sidestep out of the aisle and follow them down the carpeted lane, envious of Andy, who got to stay back.

Dear God, please help my friends not see me down here right now.

That was my biggest prayer. It was very different from the mumblings coming out of my parents' mouths, and from several other adults who came over to touch my head and pray.

"Heal her. Restore her body."

Voices shook and cracked. People sounded nervous. I was starting to get really mad. For one of the first and only Sundays since seventh grade, I was more than ready once the music ended to leave church. Why did everyone seem to know something I didn't? *Do I have cancer?*

We hadn't pulled out of the church parking lot yet, but I couldn't hold it in. My parents flashed each other a nervous look from the front seat—like their own big secret had just been busted. Andy didn't say anything.

"My Sunday school teachers knew about my colonoscopy. And they asked if I had cancer today. Isn't that weird?" I laughed. "I told them no—that's right, right?"

Mom looked back at me, then at my dad, who was focused on breaking into the line of cars also trying to exit the parking lot. My brother looked out the window, staying eerily quiet.

"Well, we don't really know," Mom finally answered. "Dr. Taormina found a mass in your colonoscopy. It might be a tumor. He's testing it to see if it's cancer."

Time stopped. The world went silent. Those weren't the words I'd expected to hear. I didn't say anything in response, but I felt my face tighten and scowl. Taken aback, disappointed, I couldn't believe not the news itself, but that I was apparently the *last* to know. It was about *my own body*, for gosh sakes! I looked out the window and said not a word the rest of the way home.

1/21/01

Mikey,

Today was odd. After church I was kind of dragged down with everyone asking me if I had cancer. I know their prayers are supposed to be a good thing, but they made me feel worse. You are just about the only one who will see the weak side of me—lucky. I'm thankful I have a friend like you to tell. In honesty, I am a little nervous. I was scared for what the doctor would find. And now I'm praying for good or okay test results. All I can do is all I ever do—pray about it. Maybe all this has come so I can be a witness to myself and others about prayer. I'm excited to start writing again. I'll pray for your upcoming semester and job hunt. Have a great week—I love you!

—Danielle

When I was just fifteen years old, I decided I wanted a job. I liked the idea of earning my own money as much as I liked getting out of the house. A public library had opened near our neighborhood, and it was within walking distance, which meant I could walk to work if I didn't have a ride. I had fond memories of the library. I loved its grand opening, where I got balloon animals, crafts, and snacks. During the summer reading program, I got free books. One afternoon, I learned they hired teenagers and applied. I was ecstatic when a lady named Gayla called me a few days later for a job interview and eventually hired me.

"Yessss!" I gladly accepted the offer.

I'd always loved books and reading. As a little girl, I got lost inside stories. I'd connect with characters who, when nobody else did, understood me. I couldn't wait to be surrounded by books all day long—or at least during a few four-hour shifts.

From my first day on the job, I knew the library was a special place. Coworkers acted like family. They hosted potlucks and remembered birthdays. They greeted me with a smile each time I walked in, oftentimes not realizing I'd just come from a house full of tension. Linda, the assistant librarian, gave us M&Ms and called them Vitamin M. Dorothy at the desk liked to joke around and was passionate about equality. My teenage coworkers like Courtney and Josh were fun and funny, and they soon became friends I hung out with outside of work.

To most people, our jobs looked boring. We spent hours peeling due-date stickers off the backs of books, reshelving novels, and memorizing the Dewey decimal system. But we liked it. Our boss, the branch librarian, Gayla, made working at the library one of the best jobs in town.

Unlike the bosses I'd heard horror stories about, Gayla was kind and nice. She wrote in nearly perfect cursive handwriting, almost always in pencil. She wore a rubber thimble over her thumb like most quilters do—a hobby she enjoyed outside of work. Her calm demeanor set a tone for the whole library. Everyone was welcome and treated with respect. She was gracious with fines when people couldn't pay. She was also forgiving of her staff. On a few occasions, I forgot she'd scheduled me to work, and it wasn't uncommon for me to run a few minutes late. But she didn't chew me out. A gentle reminder was all it took to nudge me to start arriving on time.

Dressed in pastel shirts and khakis, which matched her soft smile, her presence was inviting when I'd find myself wandering into her office each week to sit for a few minutes and talk. She taught me how to lead and stay kind under pressure. Gayla often asked about my life outside of work, genuinely interested. One time she invited some of us teens to her house for a pool party. Without yet knowing what a mentor was, I craved even a few minutes with her.

The library had become therapeutic, a book-filled sanctuary where reshelving titles and straightening up tables and chairs provided a healing consistency. So even after a really rough start to my week—with a GI appointment, a colonoscopy, and now a cancer scare—there was nowhere else I wanted to be. Plus, Tuesday nights were fun to work, not only because of the company, but because we got special jobs. Adult programs hosted in the children's area meant we could spend at least an hour of our shift fetching and rearranging tables and chairs. Although my focus was off, my body felt fine. I loved pushing around the furniture.

"There we go. They're all straight!"

We had just put the finishing touches on a set of

perfect rows when I looked up and saw Dad, and then Mom, walk into the library. My heart sank. This couldn't be good. We'd all been waiting for the doctor's call. I assumed they'd received it and not waited for me to get home. They spotted me in the back, and we met near the middle of the YA section. The Berenstain Bears and Clifford series sat on the shelves just behind me.

"Hi. What are you guys doing here?" I whispered, trying to act as if I didn't know. I looked to the side and noticed my friends staying back, confused about my parents showing up.

Mom and Dad stared at me for a second. I could tell Mom had been crying.

Finally, Dad broke the silence in a hushed library voice. "The doctor's office called with your results. The mass they found during your colonoscopy was a tumor. It's malignant."

Time stood still as I watched their eyes turn red and well with tears. Not in five years had I watched them do something with such unity. They were on the same page—clearly very sad and scared. I wrinkled my forehead. I didn't understand.

"What does 'malignant' mean?"

I had never heard the word before. In fact, I had never heard most of the words being used around me the past week. I understood "tumor" and "biopsy," but not until the doctor's appointment had I ever heard of a "colonoscopy" or "gastroenterologist." Truth be told, I'd never been taught about the "colon" and "rectum" either. I'd only known them as "intestines."

Dad cleared his throat, looked at Mom, and looked

back at me with sad eyes. "Cancer. Malignant means you have cancer, Danielle."

I thought and felt nothing. I didn't know what to do or say. Nothing in the children's books behind me had prepared me for this situation. My parents instantly wrapped their arms around me, but I felt more and more numb. The hugs were easing their own pain. I wasn't sure what I felt, if anything. I was simply stunned.

Dad cleared his throat, looked at Mom, and looked back at me with sad eyes. "Cancer. Malignant means you have cancer, Danielle."

I needed to leave, although my shift wasn't over. While I got my coat from the break room, Mom and Dad found Gayla and told her the news. I was thankful she also worked Tuesday nights.

I waved goodbye to my friends, attempting to mouth an explanation. "I'll explain everything later."

Somehow, I got home that night. (I think I drove myself, but I'm not sure.)

How many other people knew? I assumed a lot, given what had happened at church on Sunday. It was funny because once it was official that I had cancer, I really didn't care who was aware of my health—with one exception: Mike. I searched the house and found the cordless phone in my brother's room.

"Andy, can I use this?" It was a rare moment where

we actually saw each other face to face in the evening. He too stayed out of the house as much as possible and out of the way. I thought it was strange he was at home.

"Sure. Here you go." He was unusually nice to me.

I took the handset and went into my room, closing the door behind me. This required a call and not an Instant Messenger chat. I knew Mike wouldn't be expecting me, since I usually worked Tuesday nights, but I prayed he would pick up.

"Hello?"

"Hey, it's me."

"Hey . . ."

"Well, we found out what it is." I took a long pause. It was one thing to be told I had cancer, but it was another thing to tell the news to someone else.

"Yeah? What's going on?"

My voice shook. "Um, well . . . it's cancer."

The call went quiet, neither one of us knew what to say. With such a heavy heart, I wished he was in town so we could be in the same place. The hard plastic handset squished against my ear was a feeble substitute for physical human comfort, even if we were just friends.

"Wow. Okay. I'm so sorry. Are you okay?"

It wasn't a question I got asked often (yet), and I didn't know how to answer it. "Yeah, I think so. I can't really talk now. I'll call you tomorrow."

We quickly hung up, and I looked at myself in my vanity mirror. *Am I okay?* I wasn't really sure. When I'd initially heard the word *cancer*, two dads I knew of came to mind. One of them was diagnosed with pancreatic cancer and died within a few months of his diagnosis. I was friends with his kids; they were in our youth group, and it shocked us all. So sad. The other dad had a brain tumor and seemed to be healthy—he actually said hi to me at church on Sunday. It didn't seem real that I was entering their "club." Besides, I was fine and healthy, except for a little blood.

I heard the front door squeak open, and my parents greeted Nick. In major moments all throughout my life, they'd been quick to call for a pastor. A pastor came right away the day my mom's brother tragically died in a car crash and on the day her dad surprisingly died too. But never before had a minister been called over on my account. Fortunately, it was Nick. He and Leslie had become like a second set of parents to me thanks to youth camp and weekends at their place. I was actually really glad to see him.

I took a few deep breaths in front of the mirror before leaving my room to join my family. As I walked through the darkness of the hallway and made my way into the living room light, it was like a lightbulb went off in my head. In a flash, I was filled with inexplicable hope and joy.

This is really going to spice up my testimony.

It made no sense, but as I walked down the stairs, something inside my heart filled up. In one millisecond I felt numb, then scared and shocked I had cancer, yet in another, *excited*. I'd been writing to Mike as I anticipated the news, saying I hoped God could use me during my junior year. As I hugged Nick and we all gathered in a small circle to pray, the Bible stories I'd known my whole life came to mind. They were stories of people who faced daring adventures and did big things for God. Their lives weren't easy—they were full of struggles too. David faced Goliath. Esther approached the king. Joshua marched around a huge wall, and my namesake, Daniel, had almost been eaten by lions. The disciples had suffered to tell others about Jesus, and Paul wrote letters from prison. For once I could relate to suffering—Danielle had cancer!

The way I saw it, nearly all my life had been lived in a nice, suburban neighborhood where things went as planned and stayed on track. Sure, I'd faced some hardships, especially the past few years, but they were stories to keep mostly hidden and never told. The secrets about life at home couldn't be part of my testimony. I preferred to keep the truth about hating my body quiet too. But cancer—this was different. Was it ever. I could talk about cancer. There was no hiding this one. I'd found my Goliath and my lion's den.

PART 2

11

Read Job

IN A WAY, I FELT oddly prepared to get colon cancer at age seventeen. Well, sort of.

"Read Job."

I remembered first hearing the voice at Emily's house. It was clear as day. But I wasn't sure who'd spoken it, not even sure I'd technically *heard* it with my ears. But it was undeniable that *something* was with me as I wrestled with the covers in Emily's brother's top bunk bed and looked over at the glowing clock: 3:00 a.m.

I wasn't familiar with the room, having never been in it before. I was spending the night at Emily's house, and her parents had put us in her brother's room. While my younger self would have made ugly faces at the idea of sleeping in a *boy's* room, I didn't really care anymore. Truth was, I was just happy to get a sleepover, even if it meant sleeping in boy bunk beds. As I climbed to the top bunk and got cozy under dark-blue sheets, Emily and I talked over the events of the evening. We were basking in the newness of junior high and the tidal wave of excitement that flowed following our first school dance.

"Lindsay's dress was so pretty."

"Did you see that couple holding hands?"

I'd never dressed up like a woman before, nor had I been in a room full of loud music and gangly teenagers. As we'd started junior high, I slowly dropped my firm protest against *all* dresses. The handful of nice dresses I'd worn throughout elementary school were girly and cutesy, nothing like the black, tighter-fitting dresses Emily and I got to wear to our first dance. They modestly showed off our curves and budding bustlines. Emily had worn a knee-length velvet dress that sparkled. My black-and-white floor-length dress came borrowed from Kristi. But once Mom zipped up the back for me, it didn't much matter that the dress wasn't brand new—I felt pretty. For the first time in my life, I'd maybe tasted what it felt like to be a model in a magazine. With curled hair, bright makeup, and high heels, I'd now stepped into a world I'd only once dreamed of entering.

As we strode into the dance at our school, we noticed that the big overhead gym lights that normally buzzed like bees were dimmed, their slight hum overshadowed by pop songs. Laughs and squeals from girls like me who'd never felt so pretty echoed like surround sound. Wafts of Sunflowers perfume overspray billowed through the gym, masking any leftover essence of the boys' sweaty wrestling matches. Awestruck and excited, I spent most of the night glued to the painted cinderblock walls.

We didn't dance with any boys, nor did we try to

break into the circle of friends taking over the dance floor. Fact is, beyond Mom's Richard Simmons workout tapes, I'd never danced before. But dancing skills didn't matter because just attending the dance was enough. A taste of freedom. A glimpse into adolescent beauty. And it was the eve of my literally becoming a teenager.

Although I already felt like a teen, and my body looked like one, I wasn't official. This drove me crazy. I was already doing teenage girl things I'd learned about in "the talk," like dealing with periods, wearing bras, and shaving. I'd had numerous talks with Mom about everything from puberty and my body to the birds and the bees and how babies were made. As a tween, I disliked answering "Twelve" when people asked my age. I couldn't wait to proudly exclaim, "Thirteen!"

I typically woke up at home on my birthday, but since the night of the dance fell on the same night as Dad's work Christmas party, we changed our tradition: I would become a thirteen-year-old at Emily's house. It couldn't have been more perfect. I went to a dance with a friend. Mom and Dad went on a date. And I got a sleepover. In no way was I expecting a mysterious, life-changing wake-up call.

"Read Job."

I'd been sleeping soundly, but somehow the voice got me to wake up. It was haunting, as if someone was whisper-talking to me. But nobody was in the room with us, nor had anyone stepped in to wake me up. It eerily felt like one of my favorite films, *Field of Dreams*. Except the voice wasn't telling me to build a baseball field, but to wake up and, oddly enough, read the Bible.

I closed my eyes and tried to shake it off.

Maybe it's just a dream.

Pulling the covers to my chin didn't put me back to sleep. Wide awake, I couldn't rest. My senses were on high alert, as was the hair on my arms. The voice soon spoke again: *"Read Job."*

I felt crazy. An interest in faith and church had continued to snowball since Camp Shamineau, but nothing like this had ever happened to me. I wasn't sure I liked it, and I began to second-guess the voice itself.

Maybe I'm dreaming, or imagining things, or talking to myself! I hoped.

Yet deep down, I couldn't deny it, and neither could my goose bumps (which refused to recede). *Something* was in the room with me, and an inaudible voice wanted me to wake up. After a while, I obeyed.

Surely there's a Bible in here. There's got to be, I thought while surveying the dark bedroom from the top bunk.

Emily's family attended church as much as mine; it was one reason we so quickly became such good friends. She too had no choice but to spend her Sundays at church. Like Kristi's, Emily's and my rules were similar when it came to dating, clothes, makeup, and boys. And while I resented our shared rules when we met in sixth grade, after Camp Shamineau, I respected them. I had reread a lot of the Bible in the five months since camp, but the book of Job wasn't included. I also didn't recall learning about Job on the church's felt-board skits like we did with characters such as Noah, David, Joshua, and Father Abraham.

Ah, there you are.

Fortunately, I spied a bookshelf behind me and a

hardbound *Adventure Bible*. It looked just like the one I'd carried to church for years. I clicked on the bendy desk light clipped to the wooden bedpost. Rubbing my tired eyes, I became thankful for years of Bible drills and turned right to Job 1:1.

"In the land of Uz there lived a man whose name was Job. This man was blameless and upright; he feared God and shunned evil."

Uz made me think of Oz, and I wondered if a tornado, yellow-brick road, and Wicked Witch would soon be part of the story. The next few verses explained what kind of person Job was—a husband and dad, a business owner, and someone who loved God and hated evil. I instantly liked him. I kept reading.

"One day the angels came to present themselves before the Lord, and Satan also came with them. The Lord said to Satan, 'Where have you come from?' Satan answered the Lord, 'From roaming throughout the earth, going back and forth on it.' Then the Lord said to Satan, 'Have you considered my servant Job? There is no one on earth like him; he is blameless and upright, a man who fears God and shuns evil'" (Job 1:6–7).

My eyebrows furrowed—God recommended Job to Satan? God, someone I'd been taught was only good and holy, let Satan roam the earth? And mess with people?

It didn't add up, nor did it make sense. I kept reading.

"So Satan went out from the presence of the Lord and afflicted Job with painful sores from the soles of his feet to the crown of his head" (Job 2:7).

God let Satan physically hurt Job? Wow, now that was horrible. If Uz was like Oz, it would have been

My eyebrows furrowed—God recommended Job to Satan?

like God letting the Wicked Witch haunt and taunt Dorothy tirelessly. What kind of God would allow that? I kept reading.

The story went from bad to worse—Job ended up losing family, health, and all his money. He was standing at gravesites mourning his kids, all because God let Satan test him. My mind couldn't comprehend how or why God would allow something so horrible to take place. I also didn't understand why a still, small voice woke me up to read this on my thirteenth birthday.

From three to four to five o'clock, I read every word of Job's story. I couldn't put it down, and somehow my eyes weren't heavy. I understood why Job's wife told him to curse God. Their situation seemed so unfair. I didn't blame his friends for offering him awful advice. I probably would have said the same things to him too. Job's faith didn't seem to line up with his situation. Job loved and served God, and look where that got him! Yet I kept reading because the quiet voice didn't want me to stop. And I was really hoping for a happy ending.

It ended up being an extremely long book, forty-two chapters in all. But not till the final chapters did the story finally turn around. First, God spoke and reminded Job and his friends of who He was. I liked God's points—He was the creator of the world, He was in charge, and He decided what was good. I was surprised to read that Job didn't give up his faith.

Despite every foul thing that happened to him, Job remained a righteous man. At the end of the story, it got really good. God restored Job's health, business, and family, and then some. Job's replenished fortunes were *doubled*. His friends and family came over, and together they ate. As the story goes, "So the LORD blessed Job in the second half of his life even more than in the beginning" (Job 42:12 NLT).

When I turned the page and Psalm 1 appeared, I closed the Bible, put it back on the shelf, clicked off the light, and pulled the sheets to my face. I should have been tired, but I wasn't. It was as if every cell in my body, every thought in my brain, was awake. I had more questions than answers about the story, as well as what was happening to me.

Why did God allow Satan to test Job? How did Job survive all that? Was the voice I heard God? And if the voice was God, why did He wake me at three o'clock to read about suffering *on my thirteenth birthday?*

I had no answers, but I did know one thing—turning thirteen already was life-changing. Although it spooked me at first, I felt peace when the still, small voice kept talking to me, which would become a regular thing.

By the time the sunrise pierced through the dark curtains, I was already awake.

"Happy birthday!"

The rays of light woke up Emily, who of course had no idea what had just happened. I rolled over, faked a yawn, and pretended to stretch my arms so it appeared I'd also been sleeping. I wasn't ready to tell her, or anyone, about the voice and reading Job. It was too strange.

"Thank...you!" I replied in a scratchy voice. Although I'd been awake, I hadn't spoken. As we both came to life under warm and cozy blankets, I felt the chill of the air leak in. It felt like my birthday, and it looked like it too. I could see colorful, twinkling Christmas lights lining neighbors' houses. I imagined tiny, frosty snowflakes were stuck to the windows just behind the drawn curtains too.

"We're here to get our birthday girl!" Mom's voice broke the silence as I heard Emily's front door swing open. I'd assumed they felt a little bad when I didn't wake up at home on my thirteenth, and that was why they'd come to retrieve me so early. Most other days, I would have begged to stay at Emily's house all day long, but since it was my birthday, I was ready for home. Although it was tension filled, I wanted to be with my family and experience my first day of teenage life with them. Soon the bedroom door cracked open, and all four parents peeked in.

"Happy birthdayyy!" they chimed in unison. It wasn't a scene I could ever have dreamed up. Four smiling parents peering into a boy's room as I buried myself under blankets and lay on a top bunk. Although unexpected, it was perfect. The morning had already started off weird. Once I saw them, I didn't hesitate to jump off the bed, grab my overnight bag, and give Emily a hug goodbye.

"How was last night?" my parents asked on the short drive home.

I filled them in on most everything I could remember about the music, the parents who chaperoned, and the awkwardness of watching people my age learn how to dance. Dad referred to dancing as "cutting a rug" and thoroughly cracked himself up. Mom seemed glad I'd truly had a fun time. I told them everything they wanted to know about the dance and the sleepover at Emily's. But I didn't mention my three o'clock mystery—the inexplicable voice and Bible lesson. In fact, for years I didn't tell anyone about that morning. But I never forgot it.

Curiously, the evening my parents stood in the library and told me flat out I had cancer, the memory from four years prior, of my thirteenth birthday, flooded back. When I looked for answers . . . how, God? And *why?* I could think of nothing other than Job's story.

Facing one of the most unlikely cancer cases, a less than 1 percent chance of occurrence, had God oddly seen fit to prepare me for something as wild as this? Me—the volleyball player and Christian girl—facing a life-threatening disease at age seventeen? It made no sense until I went back to Job, chapter 1, and reread another unlikely story.

12

The Reveal

WHEN YOU'RE A TEENAGER GROWING up in a suburban home like mine, the world is set up to help
you thrive. (But I didn't fully realize it at the time.) Want
to learn how to drive? There's a program for that—driver's ed—assuming your dad can't teach you. Interested in
going to college? Find a tutor, teacher, or standardized
test guide, *stat*. Need a group of friends? There are clubs,
groups, and mentors galore. But as a seventeen-year-old
trying to figure out how to survive cancer, especially one
that mostly afflicts people my grandparents' ages, there
wasn't exactly a step-by-step guide. And that was why the
morning after I received the most dramatic, life-changing news ever, "You have cancer," I got up, took a shower,
got dressed, and drove to school. I even got away with
skipping breakfast.

It seemed best to make it a "normal" day because I
didn't know what else to do. I wasn't going to lie in my

bed and sulk. I had no framework for what having cancer even meant, and I was blissfully unaware of its gravity—well, almost. I didn't want to let myself think about it, so I didn't. But once I'd made it into the high school building and slid into a hard plastic chair, everything hit. The bell ringing might have kicked off class lectures across the rest of the building, but it fired a torpedo of high-wire anxiety all through me.

Yesterday I did this, but I was sitting here with cancer. I have cancer inside my body right now? How long have I had it? Where did it come from? Can other people tell?

I'd robotically pulled out my textbook, pencil, and paper as my math teacher's lecture began, yet my paper stayed blank as an unfamiliar rush of panic raced through me. My eyes bounced from wall poster to wall poster in hope of finding a worthy distraction.

Armpits sweating, heart racing. I felt so totally alienated from my attentive, note-taking classmates. They were suddenly so different, although they had no idea.

I was literally sitting on a tumor that, if it didn't get removed, would kill me. They were just trying to get through math class.

The bell rang, and after I packed up my stuff, I fairly floated back into the hallway. It felt like an invisible tranquilizer dart had been fired into me. My body still worked. I could walk down the stairs and classrooms, sure, but my mind was in a different place. Especially when I sat down in history. I took out another blank notebook page in preparation to take notes. But before I knew it, the bell rang, and the page beneath me was once again blank. Though the lecture had gotten me thinking: was *I* about to become history? Would my life soon be a lost mini-civilization to study? A new, unwieldy pressure was overwhelming.

I told a handful of teachers my news that day. When I mentioned my cancer to my Spanish teacher, whom I'd always felt close to, she replied empathetically, "Oh my gosh! I'm so sorry—are you okay? Don't worry about this class at all!"

Her words brought comfort, but also a new reality.

I was literally sitting on a tumor that, if it didn't get removed, would kill me. They were just trying to get through math class.

School. Graduation. I hadn't even thought about how getting cancer would impact my grades. My GPA sat close to a 4.0, and I had college prep tests coming up. I wanted to enroll in Mike and Scott's university, and I was on track to join them in a little over a year.

Is cancer going to stop me from graduating on time?

It was a fear nearly deeper than dying. Not only did I prefer to walk across the stage in a cap and gown alongside my friends, but the thought of graduating with the class one year younger than me, with Andy, was absolutely terrifying. Once the final dismissal bell rang, I bolted from class. I needed to go home.

Quickly, I stopped by my locker to pack books, although I was in no shape to study or do homework. I figured that even if my long-recurring high school dream was to come true—I'd show up wholly unprepared for a test—dealing with cancer had already become a way bigger problem. As I began to walk the hallways and leave school, I felt a little bad I hadn't told my friends about my cancer yet. Honestly, I didn't know what to say. I didn't understand what having cancer *really* meant yet. My parents were the ones dealing with phone calls and scheduling more doctor's appointments. I had no clue what came next.

The burst of arctic January air blasting my face was a bracing, much-needed moment. Although it was cold, my clenched jaw relaxed. I'd made it through a full day of school with the knowledge: I had cancer. As I walked down the sidewalk past the modular classrooms, I saw a friendly, familiar face—my friend Adam. We'd met in seventh grade and became fast friends. He was happy and always filled our school hallways with enthusiasm. Although we rarely hung out outside of school, Adam was also really strong in his faith, and we co-led several Christian clubs and events like See You at the Pole. It was nice to not feel like the only junior passionate about God.

Tired and exhausted, I wanted to do nothing more than collapse on the couch and watch cable TV. But as I saw Adam walking toward me, I felt the still, small voice challenge me to say something.

"Hey, Adam, can I tell you something? I haven't told anyone else today. Um, can you keep it quiet?"

He nodded to show he was listening and stepped in closer.

I fumbled for the words. Telling a friend I had cancer was a lot harder than telling adults. "Um, so, I've got cancer. I have a tumor in my intestines. I had a thing at the hospital last weekend, and the doctor found it. I'm not sure what will happen, but I'll probably need to have surgery and will be gone for a few weeks."

He basically got the same spiel as my teachers, but his response was much different. Before I knew it, he wrapped me in a big hug. I wasn't sure what to say, and neither was he. As we walked away, I was glad I had told him. No doubt. He'd pray for me.

I finally made it to my car and pulled into the line of others trying to leave the parking lot. As I looked back out of my rearview mirror at the school building, I wondered how and when I would tell more of my friends. I knew they needed to know, and they eventually would find out. I figured I had a few more days to break the news, but I was wrong. Little did I know that I wouldn't be back the next day so I could tell them—or for any of the other school days. In fact, I wouldn't be back to school for the rest of the semester. Once I got home, my mom filled me in on the plan. She and Dad took care of notifying school administration. As it turned out, fighting cancer needed all my time.

1/25/01
Mikey,
This week has drained me—my strength, smiles, and sleep—altogether. I'm not saying they are totally gone, but just for tonight. I'm scared and nervous. My big prayers are that the cancer hasn't spread. I guess this cancer thing has made every-

one think about how life is fragile. I know it has me. Through all of this, you've been there for me. Like I told you—this is all thanks to you—in a very good way. I see it as you helped save my life—and my colon. ☺ God's going to take care of me. Love you, Mikey.

—Danielle

I hated him. Hated him. And that says a lot, since I rarely flung around the word *hate*, especially about a person. But I couldn't help but storm out of the general surgeon's office with near fumes radiating off of me, mad and angry.

The days following my diagnosis went relatively well, or so I thought. I handled having cancer the best I knew how, and I felt optimistic about getting rid of it.

At first, I wasn't crying or complaining. I wasn't really too scared either. I knew the adults were terrified. I could see it in their eyes.

But to me, cancer was just a major inconvenience, at least at first.

I'd prided myself on being the kid who stayed out of doctors' offices and hospitals. But I quickly took Andy's place as I made it through a bunch of pokes and prods. I even got pushed through big equipment like CT (computed tomography, ugh) scanners and PET (positron emission tomography) scan machines. I quickly learned how to "Breathe in. Hold . . . Breathe" and received the stuff wherein once it gets pushed into the IV tube, it feels like you've just peed. Despite the medical culture shock, I was staying positive. But after meeting with the first surgeon who said he could remove my tumor, I wasn't so confident.

Several people in suburbia had recommended the guy, which, where we were from, was like gold. We valued word-of-mouth recommendations; it came with being a good neighbor. We'd found my gastroenterologist by asking around, and we assumed this surgeon would be a good fit too. But after only a few minutes in his paneled office, I began to have my doubts. Not only was his ego big, but I didn't feel comfortable with his plan. He wanted to operate by going through my rectum and then somehow extracting my tumor in pieces. As much as I liked the sound of no scars or major cutting, it didn't feel right. This was *can*cer we were dealing with, and from my understanding of the colonoscopy report, my tumor was pretty good sized. Plus, I was a seventeen-year-old female dealing with colorectal cancer. I wasn't an everyday, random surgery case. Even I knew that much.

My parents felt uneasy too. They shifted awkwardly in the uncomfortable exam room that we had all crammed ourselves into. But based on the arrogance rolling off of him, I doubted my voice would be heard. He was barely looking at me anyway, focusing mainly on Mom and Dad.

I don't like your plan . . . the one where you're going to go into my rear and pull out my tumor.

The thought was trapped inside my mind. And while I thought the visit was bad, I had no idea it was about to get much worse.

"I need to take a look."

Of course he did. I'd been prepared for this kind of moment on the way to the GI's office, but somehow it hadn't registered that the surgeon would need to do a rectal exam too. I held my breath, rolled my fingers into a fist, and gritted my teeth. His oblivion to how I felt made it even worse. I was hopeful the nurse could pick up my disdain when she handed me another backless gown and gave me the same instructions: "Waist down."

Anger, shame, and anguish flooded in as I stepped out of my jeans and followed instructions. I didn't want him touching, cutting, or even looking at my body, but I didn't have a say or choice, once again. I wanted to scream, "No, you can't take a look," but I knew by now that noncompliance wasn't an option. My head understood doctors were requesting to do the exams for medical purposes, but my heart didn't care. Nothing made me feel any better leading up to, during, or after the violating moment. Especially since it was with a man I'd never met.

I didn't want him touching, cutting, or even looking at my body, but I didn't have a say or choice, once again.

Unlike Dr. Taormina, the arrogant doctor lacked compassion. He didn't communicate what he was doing, nor was he gentle. Since his goal was "getting a good look at the tumor," his movements felt rough and aggressive. He wasn't aware how much applying pressure hurt, or that the exam lasted a little longer than I felt was needed. Had I more guts and less shock, I might have cracked a joke like, "Now that will be five dollars for admission." But by the time his rubber gloves snapped off and landed in the bottom of a small lined trash can, my clothes were back on, and I stormed out, never to look back again. I wasn't interested in a follow-up appointment or further conversations.

Disgusted. Hurt. Enraged. I felt so many things in the parking lot. I didn't care if he was the best surgeon in the city; I didn't want him operating on me. I didn't want another man like him ever touching me again.

"He is NOT going to be my doctor!" I insisted. In a rare and unique move, I'd found my (loud) voice. No doctor with that level of arrogance and incompetence was going to work on me. No man like him would ever see me waist down again. If it was between him operating or no surgery at all, I would choose no surgery, fully aware of what it meant for the tumor to stay.

"We have one more appointment tomorrow with a colorectal surgeon," Dad offered in a calm reply. "Dr. Taormina recommended him. His name's Dr. Connor. Maybe you'll like him."

I'm not sure who prayed harder for the visit with Dr. Connor to go well—them or me.

By the time Dr. Connor walked into his exam room to greet my parents and me, I felt like I'd been facing cancer for years. In truth, technically, it had only been a few days. Yet a heaviness hung over us, a blanket of fear.

Was I really facing colon cancer at age seventeen? In real life? We were going through the motions, but it was hard to embrace reality.

Yet reality was what led to a hopeful colorectal surgeon visit, which I liked saying much more than "proctologist." As I stared up at the man, who stood at least six foot five, I wondered the same thing about him as I did my GI.

What on earth made you want to go into this field?

I swallowed my question and sat quietly on another sheet of crinkled paper as Dr. Connor thumbed through my chart. It was getting thick already. Peering through his glasses to read over my reports, he gave a look I'd come to expect, as well as the comment. "You're awfully young for colon cancer."

I'd learned to simply smile and nod. What else was I going to say? "Lucky me"?

Dr. Connor began talking, mostly to my parents, although he occasionally paused and looked my way. I was used to doctors avoiding conversations with me. I figured since I was technically a minor, my parents were ultimately in charge. And really, I didn't mind. I appreciated that Mom and Dad were taking care of making appointments and navigating the hospital's parking garages. They were the ones on the phone with insurance companies and paying the bills. My job was just to get on the "medical carousel," as I called it (a.k.a. "get in the car and go").

Though I felt weary from meeting so many new doctors, Dr. Connor did seem different. He spoke slowly and gently, and despite his height, he was approachable and nonthreatening. His silver hair gave me comfort; his experience quickly became clear. Unlike the other doc, who did general surgery, Dr. Connor worked only on the digestive system. He spoke slowly, humbly, and used pen-and-paper sketches to explain his plan.

"We'll make the incision here." He drew down the middle of an illustrated abdomen. And although his plan apparently involved a long, vertical abdominal scar, my actual chest didn't tense up when I saw the sketch. His intention to move my organs out of the way, find my tumor, and remove not only the section of colon with the tumor in it, but "margins," as he called them, sounded smart. We all agreed, we needed to make sure the cancer hadn't traveled anywhere else. For once, I had a strange peace.

But then he threw a curveball. "There is a chance I'll need to do an ostomy."

We had made it through the big stuff, and I'd decided privately in my heart—he was the one. This is the guy! But then he dropped the bomb. Because my tumor was so close to the rectum, there was a chance I'd need a permanent ostomy—meaning a bag would hang from my stomach, and I'd never go poop "normally" again. I shook my head as the words came out of his mouth.

"No. I am not getting the bag. Do not give me the bag. Whatever you do—no."

Up until this point, I'd been quiet and compliant. I would even dare to say I liked the guy. But when I heard that a poop bag could possibly hang from my stomach, forever, it brought back every insecurity and fear. No longer was I a strong seventeen-year-old female sitting on crinkly paper and coping relatively well with the shocking case of colon cancer. In the moment I was notified that I might need an ostomy, I regressed to the embarrassed, insecure, tween fighting her mom in the middle of a Walmart toilet paper aisle.

Just dealing with colon cancer, and all the unavoidable potty talk that came with it, was a stretch for me. Nearly overnight, my poop had gone from a subject I discussed with *no* one to seemingly everybody's business. And while I wanted to be more mature, and I knew beauty came from the inside, I couldn't fathom life with an ostomy. It was devastating.

"I beg you—do not do that to me."

"I will see what I can do, but no promises."

I'd never begun praying so quickly, and so fervently, for anything in my life. Despite the ostomy shock wave, by the end of the consult with Dr. Connor, I knew we'd met the right guy. I figured he too would ask to "take a look" to close out an otherwise pleasant visit and I was right. His rectal exam felt just as rude and unpleasant as the others, but I didn't get redressed feeling quite as hopeless.

Upon getting diagnosed with cancer, I'd made sure to call and tell a few people personally. I called Kristi, who was in her dorm room at college. I also let Emily know a day or so after I found out. Courtney, my friend from the church and library, also had to know. But outside of a handful of friends, and still before the social media era, I let news of my cancer spread naturally. Andy carried updates to our teachers at school when they'd ask, although he quickly became tired of the "Danielle updates."

"I told them you died," he'd semi-joke after explaining how annoying it felt to keep getting questions about me. And while I knew it was his way of handling the awkwardness, it was a reminder that as teenagers, we couldn't quite comprehend cancer's seriousness. Watching Andy deal with it opened my eyes to the reality that cancer wasn't just affecting me. Cancer affected our entire family, our entire community. For those who liked to cook, this meant good things. Meals began to show up as friends from Sunday school and the ladies from the library heard our news. They carried in trays of lasagna and salad, plus hearty pots of chicken and noodles, to remove the nightly burden of dinnertime.

As a lot of adults stepped in to help my parents, and Andy had his friends, Mike comforted me. The weekend following my diagnosis, he came home and took me to the high school to cheer on his sister and the rest of the girls' basketball team. The rustling sound of cheerleaders' pom-poms and the loud whistles blown by referees was a nice break to the soundtrack of cancer. Although technically broken up, I didn't have to ask Mike in the days that followed my diagnosis, "Will you come home?" It was a no-brainer.

The sound of his car coming down the street and the sight of his blue eyes once he stepped out melted my heart. My feelings about him hadn't gone away, and I'd been praying that maybe, hopefully, he'd feel the same way. Our relationship had been built on more than initial attractions. We were each other's types in our hearts. A few hours later, while leaving the game, he grabbed my hand to pull me close. No words were needed: we were instantly back together.

I both was and wasn't surprised that cancer didn't scare him away. Had he chosen to stay at school and keep his distance, I would have understood. Yet as my own cancer story began, I'd learn his experiences with it. When his aunt was diagnosed with advanced breast cancer, he'd rallied to support her alongside his family. She was in remission (a.k.a. cancer free), and he assumed I'd get there too.

"I prayed for God to heal you," he began writing in our journals. We both believed He would.

Because I was seventeen, doctors moved quickly. Surgery got scheduled within days, and before I knew it, friends and family filled my house with a nervous energy on the eve of my major operation. None of us knew what to expect. Unlike Mike's family, nobody in my immediate or extended family had gone through anything quite like this (especially colon cancer). Same with my friends.

I was hungry and displeased after a presurgical two-day fast and another colon prep. As for the adults? They seemed lost, so they decided to pray. Ever since the Sunday at the altar, many had put their hands on me and asked God for healing. I tried to politely smile, hiding my discomfort. As they prayed, I slipped in my own silent request. *God, get this over with so I can go back to my life.* Somehow that night, I feel asleep.

My alarm pierced the silence of my bedroom, pushing me out of bed and into the car as Dad backed out of the garage. It was still dark, and I made sure Andy knew I deserved a thank-you for getting him out of school, even if it meant waking up early. The hospital was located down the street from the Plaza, which was motivating to see. I dreamed of the day I wouldn't need to think about cancer but could simply stroll around the fountains hand in hand with Mike again, just like we did on our first date. Both of us were beaming despite the cancer, glad to be back together again. I hoped to see him soon.

Checking into the hospital involved a pattern to which I'd quickly become familiar. Take clipboard from attendant. Sign clipboard. Sit in chair. Wait. Stand up. Receive more papers from desk clerk. Fill those out. Sit back down. Visit a new clerk at a private desk. Answer more questions. Get a plastic ID bracelet. Wait for person wearing scrubs to call my name. Follow them. Strip. Slide on a backless gown. Wait my turn on the carousel. I knew the drill.

By the time I made it to the pre-op room, I was ready to get on with the surgery.

"Can you tell me your name and your birthday?" hospital staff kept asking. I assumed this was to make extra sure they didn't remove a section of colon from the wrong patient. Trying to sit still and not fidget, I was both cold and uncomfortable. I never turned down the offer of another warm blanket. The curtain-lined area where I waited was tiny, but Mom, Dad, and Andy crowded in. Pastor Nick came with them too, so he could pray one more time. While I appreciated the gesture, I'd been around so many people praying for me, I actually stopped listening. Prayer was good, but it had become overwhelming.

"We're here to take you back!"

Eventually, two ladies wearing puffy blue covers over their hair and shoes came to roll me into surgery. I waved goodbye to my family again, knowing they'd be spending the next several hours with friends who came to sit with them and sip free, dank hospital coffee. Except for Andy—he'd be drinking Cherry Coke.

As attendants steered my bed down white hospital hallways, they didn't say much, but they did give pitiful smiles, the same ones I got from most people who discovered my diagnosis and age. Bumping elbows opened two big doors that swung into a large, markedly cold room with bright lamps and a shiny stainless-steel table surrounded by metal trays. My memory of sliding over onto the operating table is vague because the next thing I knew, I was looking up and seeing Mike and his mom walking down another white hallway as new attendants wheeled me into my room.

Still groggy, I didn't notice much besides the TV up high, a room-dividing curtain, and a whiteboard on the wall in front of me. As the anesthesia eventually wore off, I saw colorful flower arrangements, gifts, and balloons along the windowsill. Courtney taped posters on the walls saying "Jamaica or Bust" to motivate me to get better. Neither of us wanted cancer to ruin our summer mission trip plans.

I felt very loved by the multitudes of people who sent gifts, called, and stopped by to visit, but I also felt fuzzy, foggy, and like I'd been hit by a truck. For the first few days, really good pain relievers largely masked surgery's sting, but they couldn't numb the discomfort from a nasty NG (nasogastric) tube running down through my nose into my stomach to suck out acid into a bucket hanging on the IV pole. It was horribly uncomfortable, not to mention gross. Gauze and white padding wrapped my stomach. Plastic tubes pumped clear liquids into me, and other tubes collected my pee. Annoying cuffs around my legs kept inflating and deflating. Helpless yet optimistic, I was ready to get back to teenage living.

When Dr. Connor walked into the room to check on me, my anticipation skyrocketed. I'd peeked under the sheets, but my stomach was bandaged so tightly, I couldn't see anything.

"Could you do it?" I asked with every ounce of hope I could find.

His smile gave away the answer, and it was all I needed. No ostomy.

2-4-01

Dear Danielle,

I am so joyful on the inside, so incredibly joyful, no one can even imagine. I prayed so hard that God would keep you here. I was scared up until I went into your hospital room and we talked. I don't remember what either of us said, but I feel better. Despite the tube coming out of your nose, you're still cute as ever. I've enjoyed spending my weekend at the hospital with you. I wouldn't have it any other way—except for you to be better. I'm still a little shady to the whole reason for this, but I know there is one, and it's going to be for the good of everyone. I prayed so hard that God would make you better. I don't want to lose my best friend. Thank you for allowing me to stay by your side and take care of you, just as much as your parents. That meant so much. I LOVE YOU!

—Michael

13

Shackles

IT FELT RUDELY IRONIC, IF I was being honest. My overarching off-limits subject, bathroom habits, had become woven into nearly every conversation.

How did I get here? I repeatedly asked myself during the weeklong hospital stay.

What do I believe about true beauty now?

Can I accept my newly scarred body?

Where is my faith?

These were questions without quick answers. They didn't come when my room was full of visitors. They also didn't come as Andy fed me ice chips with a spoon or when Mike pulled up a chair to read the Psalms to me. They came in the darkness of night, amid the distinctive sounds of nurses' rubber soles squeaking during midnight rounds. They were questions that hovered over IV poles and machines working hard to stabilize me.

"The pathology report indicates it's stage 3."

We'd been waiting for this news, and a few days after surgery, it came. Based on what looked like a disappointing conversation between Dad and Dr. Connor in the hallway, I gathered stage 3 wasn't good, or at least not what we wanted.

I'd taken basic science courses and vaguely understood how cells and genes worked. Dad tried to explain the pathology report.

"There was cancer in some of your lymph nodes Dr. Connor removed, and those lymph nodes travel up and down the body." Dad didn't have to say it. I quickly understood. If cancer was in my lymph system, it could be anywhere. I would have been told "It's stage 1 or stage 2" if the cancer hadn't gone anywhere else, like the lymph nodes. But "stage 3" meant the cancer had started to travel. Stage 4: it jumped from one organ to another. Fortunately, mine hadn't jumped, yet both stages 3 and 4 meant advanced cancer.

For the first time, I began to feel a little scared. I wasn't dealing with a minor illness like the cold or an annoying bug like the flu. I began to understand advanced cancer equaled a life-threatening disease.

If we didn't do anything to treat the cancer, I could die. It was a bit more serious than what I'd led my teachers, friends—and myself—to believe.

Things were heavy. There was no hiding it. "Is my daughter going to die?" My parents never vocalized their fears, but I knew they existed. How could they not? The chronic tension set the stage, however, for funny moments to become downright hilarious. So on the rare occasions we found something to laugh about, the time felt even more precious.

I had only been home for one day. Doctors had released me with instructions to "take it slow." I was following orders: nibbling on applesauce, eating canned pears, not moving quickly. But either I overdid it or my body simply cried out it needed more healing.

I wasn't dealing with a minor illness like the cold or an annoying bug like the flu. I began to understand advanced cancer equaled a life-threatening disease.

After a sudden urge to use the restroom, I shockingly saw a very familiar sight. Blood. More than any time before the surgery.

"Mooooooom!" I hollered in a panic.

I'd learned by now not to hide, and she rushed in just in time. My face white and pale, I suddenly felt very thirsty. After leaning my head against the wall, next thing I knew, Andy was carrying me to my bed like a lifeguard rescue. He lay me down, and Mom dialed 911, not leaving my side. There was a fear and panic in her eyes, as well as her voice, I'd never seen or heard. It was a frightful scene, one that became even more dramatic as Dad rushed in.

"What are you doing?" Andy yelled out. "Get a towel!"

I'd been out of it, but my eyes shot open. Right before me, in the doorframe of my bedroom, stood my soaking-wet father—fully naked.

"You yelled, 'We lost her!'" he said, not realizing Mom meant I'd *fainted*, not died. He stood there for a few more seconds until finally leaving the room to follow Andy's advice to towel up.

A few minutes later, several guys with ER stenciled on their backs lifted me off my bed and onto a stretcher, which they wheeled into an ambulance parked in our neighborhood street. Fortunately, Dad got dressed, and as the ambulance pulled away, my parents followed closely in our car. Mike picked up Andy, and they too came. Luckily, doctors believed the sudden rush of blood was normal following surgery. What a relief. As we sat around the hospital room once more, we couldn't help but laugh, warily. Seeing Dad soaking wet in nothing but his birthday suit had become the most hilarious moment along the entire cancer journey, a memory I clung to when things became grave.

Given the circumstances, I smiled as wide as I could. But it still felt incredibly odd to step onto a photographer's backdrop and take senior class pictures as a junior. Still, I understood why Mom and Dad made a special call and asked a photographer to make an exception—and quickly.

We'd met with an oncologist named Dr. Rosen, who said I needed chemotherapy and radiation since the cancer was stage 3. Fortunately, all the other tests showed the cancer hadn't yet spread to other organs. Although I was tired of meeting new doctors, I appreciated Dr. Rosen. He was soft spoken and articulate, and I could tell he was really smart. I also *loved* that his consultation didn't include a rectal exam. He even gave me a pass on wearing a patient gown, something his nurses said was a rare exception. Yet although I liked him personally, I didn't understand most of what he was saying. The drug names were long and X-y, and cancer treatment sounded complicated.

But I did have one question for him. "I'm signed up to go on a mission trip this summer to Jamaica. Do you think I can still go?"

The room went silent, which didn't feel like a good thing. Dr. Rosen's answer surprised me. "Let's get treatment started and see how you do . . . we'll see."

It wasn't a yes, but it wasn't a no. I was satisfied.

I tuned out and didn't listen to my parents' conversation. Although it was all about me, I didn't have a say. I did understand that in order to start chemo, Dr. Rosen wanted me to get a small, squarish Port-a-Cath implanted into my chest. And I came to learn the drugs he wanted me to get came with potential side effects.

"Mouth sores, vomiting, dry skin, hair loss."

"Hair loss . . ." I looked up.

It caught Mom's attention too. "Wait. She will lose her hair?"

Awkward pause. Dr. Rosen nodded his head to confirm. Yes, it was likely. In a split second, a hundred invisible daggers dug into my heart.

"Not my hair!" I don't know why, but the threat of losing my hair didn't seem real. I knew cancer patients often lost their hair, but for some reason, it didn't register it could happen to me.

Not since Dr. Connor dropped the potential ostomy bomb had I felt such deep panic and despair. Was I strong enough to face even more of my insecurities about beauty? I wasn't sure.

"Excuse me. I'll be back."

Up until this point, I'd not left any room I was asked to sit in, even when I wanted to run out kicking and screaming. I'd let doctors look at every place on my body they wanted. I'd answered every invasive question truthfully. But when I heard cancer might cost me my hair, things changed.

I found a dark enclave off a dimly lit hallway hiding cleaning supplies. With my back against the wall, I slid to the floor and hugged my knees. A yellow mop bucket full of dirty water sat across from me, a perfect picture to how I felt as the tears broke loose to stream down my face. Cancer was playing nasty now, and dirty.

The tears felt foreign, but I didn't stop them. I'd learned how to hold in my emotions, and I prided myself on not tearing up. The night I was told I had cancer, I didn't cry. Feeling postsurgery pain once the meds wore off? Not then either. But the instant I heard I might lose my hair, I lost it. It felt vain, but I couldn't stop crying. In the midst of trying to accept myself, I'd found beauty in my long, dark hair. It was something strangers often complimented. When I'd stare into the mirror and try to not hate what I saw, I'd learned to appreciate my body via my hair. The thought of losing it was devastating.

I would have stayed hidden in the hallway forever, but I knew someone would soon look for me. I found a bathroom and splashed water on my cheeks, pinching them a few times as a worthless attempt to disguise I'd been crying. Upon returning to the room, I hadn't missed anything. Dr. Rosen and my parents were still talking. Fortunately, the appointment wrapped up once I got back. Kim, Dr. Rosen's nurse who'd stood quietly in the corner during the appointment, shuffled over to slip me a handful of brochures before I walked out the door.

"Just in case," she whispered. "You never know . . . you may not need these."

"Thanks," I replied with a wimpy smile. I took the brochures home reluctantly and looked through them as my parents scrambled and called the photographer.

2/15/01

Mikey,

You've been telling me, "Don't be surprised if you lose your hair," but there was always a chance and prayer I wouldn't. Today the doctor explained I likely will, and it's hard to take. I feel like I was just starting to get up, and now another, much heavier, load has been dropped on me. I know everything will be all right, but it's getting harder. The thing about God is that it's hard to have faith. People who say Christians have the easy way out are fools! I think it would be so easy right now to become mad and bitter. I am trying my hardest, but I don't get the God thing right now. I am going to follow it because in my heart, I know it's right, and I don't see anything better to turn to. But I'm so confused. I didn't do anything. I've prayed and been faithful through this whole thing—why can't it just be over? Why don't the people who do drugs and party get this? I want to be aggravated, but then Jesus reminds me: He didn't smoke, drink, lie, or even gossip—yet He had to die. Also, my head tells me that I should tell you to move on—it's not fair of me to put you through this. My heart wants to keep you. I know you want to be with me and there for me, but it's just harder than I imagined. I love you mucho.

—Danielle

I assumed the visit with Dr. Rosen would start my chemotherapy. I was ready to get it over with ASAP. Once again I thought wrong. As it turned out, my case was so rare, our Kansas City doctors urged us to get a second opinion from a major cancer center. They wanted to ensure their recommendations lined up with the country's top research and expert opinions. So ten days after meeting Dr. Rosen, Mom, Dad, and I boarded a plane for M. D. Anderson Cancer Center in Houston. Grandma and Grandpa came into town to stay with Andy.

"Oh, that place is great. One of the best. They're supported by President Bush!"

Truth be told, I didn't care how good they were. I was ready to be done with cancer. If that meant traveling to Houston with my parents, so be it. I didn't have to like it. Although cancer put a lot of life on pause, it hadn't stopped Mom and Dad's fighting. The "discussions" were as constant as ever; in fact, they seemed to happen more. I felt bad when I heard them harshly whispering, wondering if my health was to blame. Had it done what I'd feared all along? Did it add one more stressor to our life?

Not only did I not want a week away with my parents, but I hated being even farther from Mike. I missed him. I actually missed school. I wanted to be with my friends. I was getting tired and weary, not to mention lonely. Since the end of January, my life had been a nonstop cancer fight. I wanted nothing more than to just feel normal for a few days and drop all the cancer stuff. But I quickly learned that's not how it works. Cancer, not me, controlled the show. For the next act, I needed to accept I'd be in Houston for ten days, whether I liked it or not.

"Patient four seven one two two three."

A little louder, the nurse repeated herself, but I sat still in the waiting room chair. Other patients in the waiting room looked around. Oblivious, I didn't realize the number she kept calling meant she needed *me*. Finally, after a third time, my parents realized it was our turn and jumped up.

"What is this? Why am I a number around here and not a name?" I grumbled aloud as Mom shushed me. I was so disappointed, and genuinely insulted. Is it too hard to say "Danielle"? I didn't like this new fancy way.

After the nurse took my height and weight, we followed her to a small room. Although we were sitting in a world-class exam room, I couldn't tell. They were all starting to look the same. White paint. A couple of cabinets and a sink. Medical supplies and posters hanging on the wall. And most often, a properly outdated issue of *People* magazine.

The waiting felt like hours, not only before we got called back but even after. Finally, a knock at the door broke the silence, and a youngish, dark-haired doctor who couldn't have been older than forty-five strutted in.

Oh no, not another one.

I was good at sniffing out arrogance. After meeting the general surgeon, I had no tolerance. He quickly became another crisp white coat to me who wasted no time reviewing my chart. Using the same big words as Dr. Rosen, he looked at Mom and Dad and started talking. But unlike Dr. Rosen, his bedside manner suffered. He didn't pay me too much attention.

My parents kept treating M. D. Anderson like the palace of cancer royalty. They took attentive notes and were even more over-the-top grateful for all the doctors who agreed to see me. And while they seemed to feel like it was a special place, I struggled to accept it. I missed my doctors at home, and I didn't like not being called by my name. I didn't appreciate that the doctors seemed to ignore me. And I hated what the oncologist assigned to me, I hope accidentally, said: "I've even had some patients outlive me."

As the comment slipped, I'd watched his proud lips curl and his pearly white teeth shine. He might as well have popped a collar and revved up a motorcycle.

I am going to outlive you, you jerk, I thought. *Hello . . . I'm only seventeen.*

I couldn't believe that he would say something like that—a guy in his forties thinking he'd be some kind of hero if he outlived me? Didn't he expect me to live? Wasn't that his job? Was I not a hopeful case? I'd thought all along that my cancer was curable, and everyone in Kansas City expected me to survive. Did he know something we didn't? Unfortunately, he wasn't the first, nor the last, to make a dumb comment.

I couldn't storm out of his office like I had the general surgeon's, because it would only have led to more complex hallways inside a big maze. But we eventually found our way outside the building, and my parents went to work trying to cheer me up. Dinner at Joe's Crab Shack. Shopping at the Galleria. Buying me a new hat from J.Crew (which did lighten my spirits a little—at least I would have a cover when my hair started dropping). But despite their attempts, I struggled to find a bright side. Everything felt hard and was a major hassle. Redoing my blood work and scans. Answering the same set of questions. After only a few days in Houston, I felt drained, exhausted, done.

Had Mike and Scott's master plan to drive to Houston over the weekend and be back for Monday classes unfolded, the story would have been different. Yet after mapping the fourteen-hour one-way trip, Mike decided to stay back and search for other ways to surprise me.

3-5-01

Dear Danielle,

I got down on the phone because you were upset and kept saying the doctors were telling you the one sentence I don't want to hear: it could come back. I don't want it to. I want it to be gone. I'm very thankful for you, and I don't ever want to lose you. Sometimes I think about what I might do if something did happen to you . . . it's not cool stuff. I have to tell myself God is going to take care of you. I LOVE YOU!

—Michael

Before we left Kansas City, my parents' friend Mirella stopped by to pray for me. She'd always carried a strong faith and charismatic energy. Throughout my illness, she and her husband, Dan, stopped by the hospital multiple times. They often brought a gift, such as new slippers or books. Before we left for Houston, Mirella brought over a cassette tape. I'd tossed it into my suitcase, along with an old-school Walkman I'd dug up in my closet, not giving it much thought. But one night in the hotel room when I couldn't sleep because I felt so anxious and angry, I tiptoed out of bed and found it. I looked at the label. It read "Mary Mary."

I put the tape into the Walkman, pushed Play, and soon heard a hip-hop group singing "Shackles" through the headphones and leading me through a catchy anthem that was praising God and declaring that He is big enough to remove spiritual shackles and chains off our feet. I'd never heard of Mary Mary before. I hadn't listened to much gospel music. But I liked it; it was not only a nice distraction from my feelings but a cover-up to Dad's loud snoring.

Once the song ended, it played again. Mirella had recorded it not once, but over and over again. As I listened, my beating heart slowed. I sensed the still, small voice was with me. For the remainder of our trip to Houston, once I slid under the covers, I'd listen to the song through the headphones. As a personal anthem for my trip, it reminded me to have faith. Things would get better soon. A few days later, I felt the first chain break.

I'd become a waiting room pro, but my patience had nearly run out. I'd skimmed almost all the magazines sitting on square tables. I'd sat through enough sitcom reruns, petty court shows, and boring morning show interviews to last me a lifetime. With a plane ticket for Kansas City dated one day away, I had one goal in mind. Not: survive cancer. Not: finish treatment. But: *Go home.* After one final scan, I'd be set free.

The doctors in Houston all agreed with my Kansas City docs. I needed chemotherapy *and* radiation. I was such a rare, high-risk, and unusual case, doctors wanted to treat it aggressively. Although stage 3, they treated me like I had stage 4 cancer. I didn't know exactly what that meant, but I didn't care. As long as the plan led to being with Mike, and cancer free, I was very agreeable.

Sitting in what I understood to be my final waiting room for the M. D. Anderson experience, I was delighted when a hospital worker called for me, even if he didn't use my name. I followed him and was asked to sit and wait in a different chair. I was less than thrilled to be getting a barium enema CT scan, especially since I knew what an enema did, thanks to my colonoscopy prep experiences. As I squiggled, squirmed, and tried to prepare myself, I heard the double doors open, and a squeaky cart roll in. It stopped just behind where I was sitting.

"Danielle Ripley?"

I looked back to see a young hospital staffer smiling at me and reaching for something labeled Net Note. Surprised to hear my name and not a number, I looked around, confused.

"Here you go, sweetie."

She handed me the note and kept walking, pushing her cart through the double doors. I looked down at the white envelope—it was clearly for me. Every appointment between five thirty and seven thirty was written on the back. I looked at the clock; it was close to eight. They'd barely found me. With hopeful yet hesitant curiosity, I tore open the envelope and pulled out a folded sheet of paper. It looked official, like some sort of telegram.

Relationship to Patient: Friend (boyfriend)

Message for patient: HI! I just got out of my test. I actually knew some of the stuff, so I was happy.

I woke up with the worst back pain this morning. It still hurts. I'll live though. At least it's not my knee, right? It's 9:36. You are probably in your meeting. I'm praying for you. I LOVE YOU! Have a good day. Talk to you later.

Wait, how did he? How could he? My heart nearly exploded. It was Mikey!

Apparently, on the cancer center's website, people could send patients a note. I became eternally grateful for the internet, undoing years of disliking it, as well as appreciative of the cancer center's high-tech tools. I'll admit—this was cool. What providential timing. I needed his note more than ever.

Seconds later, a hospital worker called my number, again, and I followed him to a window-lined room with another large machine. I tucked the note safely into my clothes, and it helped me get through the thirty minutes that followed. While the mammoth machine spun and whirled around me and flashbacks of prior scans rushed forth, I thought about the Net Note from Mike, who clearly loved me. I thought about the surprise gifts from my mom's Houstonian friends and the cards from strangers who barely knew me. I thought about the hotel room pillow fights with Dad after Mom went home and it was just us, the thrill of swinging a white pillowcase into his face and catching one in mine as we laughed and let off steam. I thought about my friends who yelled "Surprise!" several days later when I touched down in Kansas City and wheeled my suitcase into the living room.

Once I made it home, I was nowhere close to out of the woods. Some would say my cancer journey had just begun. But my faith was stronger than ever. I felt God was near. My shackles were coming off, and I hoped, I prayed, I'd soon be able to dance.

14

Dance

"**Y**OU'RE SO LUCKY!"

Each time someone said it—*lucky*—I snickered. Cancer was aging me . . . quickly. Adults didn't make comments about advanced-stage colon cancer equaling good fortune. But my peers saw my empty desk, missing school. They also saw me at the fun stuff—assemblies and dances. I suppose getting cancer did appear lucky. Usually, I understood their perspective. A precancer teenage life wasn't *so* far in my past. Not until I'd lived with cancer did I fully understand what it took.

I'd not seen anyone smother cocoa butter on sensitive scars or get a Port-a-Cath placed above their heart and into their chest. The sting of mouth sores and the metallic taste that followed chemo treatments was unknown, as was the nausea and the panic of watching chunks of

Out of every hard thing involving cancer, feeling rejected and isolated from my friends hurt the most.

hair swirl around a shower drain. Heck, before cancer, I never had to face the reality that my life, one day, would end. I knew my classmates had no clue, but sometimes, it was hard to remember.

For the first few months following diagnosis day, a flurry of activity kept me busy. Distracted. Yet as treatment got underway, I didn't only feel sick, but lonely. I'd been plucked out of a world, and it was going on without me. Just as I was learning a new vocabulary like the drug names involved in triple-combination chemotherapy and the pills to take for antinausea, my friends were learning too—but about trigonometry and world history. My days were full of either medicine dripping down plastic tubes into my veins or days in bed recovering. My classmates' days were still full of dismissal bells, slamming lockers, major tests, and snow days. I knew they had no concept of cancer, but I did get sad when so few people seemed to care.

Out of every hard thing involving cancer, feeling rejected and isolated from my friends hurt the most. I didn't want to voice my disappointment, though, because I understood why they stayed away.

Cancer was scary, for one. Plus, there were other things in life going on. Why sit and watch me lie on a couch when there's bowling, movies, and trying out our suburb's new chain restaurants? I couldn't swim in the germ-tainted lake water once the weather warmed up or join jogs around the neighborhood. I knew my body couldn't do the "normal" teenage things, but it didn't make the absence of an invitation easy to shake off. I'd become big news and received lots of concern and visitors while in the hospital for surgery. Yet as treatment wore on and people got busy, the hype was over, and I was forgotten. Well, mostly.

Some of my teachers rallied my classmates to make encouraging posters that representatives from the National Honor Society delivered. My friends in the Christian clubs I led sent a Get Well Soon poster too. Courtney had seen it all. She was working at the library when my parents told me I had cancer. Not only did she make Jamaica or Bust signs for my hospital room, but once I got discharged, she visited me several times each week. Although our dreams of going to Jamaica eventually did go bust (my doctors felt my immune system was too compromised to travel 1,700 miles to build houses in a third-world country), Courtney kept my hopes high. On nights I felt up to it, she'd pick me up and drive us to youth group or Taco Bell. It was a welcome reminder that I was only seventeen.

Emily also came around a lot. I couldn't imagine life without her. Since sixth grade we'd been nearly inseparable, and cancer didn't stop that. Em called most nights and came by the house. She wrote me a poem to which she glued pictures of us from when we first met. She too had a boyfriend, and we filled each other in on our latest relationship news. Thanks to Em, I sort of knew what happened at school—namely, the hookups and breakups.

And then, of course, there was Mike. Around four o'clock, he became the highlight of my day. After spending most of the afternoon watching reality TV, I'd walk down the driveway to fetch the mail and then slowly make my way back inside and downstairs to our computer. The daily crossword puzzle on Yahoo! was always my first stop. Despite getting a lot of practice, I needed the checker to help me fill in the blanks every time. I'd work on the puzzle while logged into Instant Messenger, waiting for a little dot to show me Mike had logged on too. Most of the time, he appeared after his last class of the day and sent a chat to say hello. For hours, we'd flirt back and forth and count down the days until the weekend. Ever since the night at the basketball game when we got back together, he came home every Friday. I felt guilty that I was taking away his college experience, but he reassured me it was what he wanted. As the late afternoon turned into evening, more friends logged on. Sometimes they'd send a quick chat to see how I was feeling. Each time they did, I treasured it.

Overall, the majority of my classmates didn't know how to support me, but the adults sure did. Encouraging letters in the mail and get-well gifts got delivered daily. Pajama pants. Fuzzy socks. Lotions and lip balm. All kinds of comfort items. Church newsletters from all over (even ones I didn't attend) included prayer needs lists and, without fail, contained my name. Hot meals from both the church and the library ladies kept coming.

I was told someone sent my name to the pope asking for special prayers, and my jaw hit the floor when a signed photo from President George W. Bush showed up in our mailbox. I was humbled, and in awe, of so many people hearing about my cancer and wanting to help.

It felt strange, this whole cancer thing, as it brought roundabout answers to prayers I both did and didn't say.

Did I actually pray for this to happen?

I couldn't help but wonder, and it felt a little ironic. Shortly before my junior year had begun, I'd begged my dad to enroll me in a small, private Christian school. I'd already noticed my classmates changing; I felt odd and out of place with my strong faith. Few others had chosen to engrave a Bible verse on their class rings. But 1 Timothy 4:12 guided me: "Don't let anyone look down on you because you are young, but set an example for the believers in speech, in conduct, in love, in faith and in purity." Although my closest friends didn't drink, a lot of others did. Couples were hooking up. Drugs and alcohol made their way into some parties. As much as I liked my friends and community, I wanted out.

Dad hadn't gone for my pitch, and I decided I'd make the best of it. In my earliest journals to Mike at the beginning of the school year, I wrote about my hopes for the year. I wanted to love my classmates well, pray for them, and find opportunities to share Jesus. Yet attending school, especially with my boyfriend so far away, was hard. When a nice gray-haired woman named Mrs. Black knocked on our front door and introduced herself as my "homebound" teacher, it sure felt like *God* had been listening (or reading). A major illness qualified me for the school district's program that kept me enrolled in my classes but allowed me to take them from home and not at the school.

A retired PE teacher who wore sneakers and always brought a big smile, Mrs. Black helped make school at home, well, fun. She liked to laugh, and I enjoyed her company. She also seemed to enjoy mine. Each week, we'd spend a few hours at the dining room table going over the assignments she had picked up from my teachers. Her role wasn't only to courier classwork to and from my house and the school, but to tutor me as needed. Based on the worksheets and assignments coming home, though, we both knew my teachers were taking it *very* easy on me. I assumed they figured cancer was teaching me *plenty* of important things.

Mrs. Black couldn't have been more awesome. My teachers, and the entire administration, were so graceful and understanding. Gayla let me keep my job and come to work when I felt like it. I daily received messages from a grandparent, aunt, uncle, or church friend that said they were praying for me. And while it felt like an army-sized group of people was helping my family and me fight cancer, a special group of people went above and beyond: my nurses.

Nurse Lori set a high bar the day I went in for my first colonoscopy. She'd looked me in the eyes, a scared seventeen-year-old unaware of what was happening and reassured me: she wasn't leaving. I knew her compassion went above and beyond her job. But what I didn't realize was she'd be the first of many.

As surgeries, chemotherapy, and radiation appointments began, I met a few doctors and a fleet of nurses. There were nurses in the ER, nurses on the hospital floors, nurses helping me get changed, and even nurses whose job it was to witness or chaperone doctors doing rectal exams on me.

They were all different in personality, role, and color or pattern of scrubs, but a common thread unified them all. They were kind. They were gentle. And they asked a lot of questions. Every nurse in every hospital had one goal: to help me feel better.

My first day of chemo could have been written off as horrible. The infusion took forever, and then I spent most of the night vomiting. But a nurse-filled entourage had all stopped by; they'd flocked by my side at some point during the day. I met Cindy and Cindy, Val, Trisha, and Toni. By the end of the infusion, I wasn't only smiling, but I didn't mind coming back. One special nurse made it her goal for me to feel that way about treatment each time, Nurse Kim.

The clinic hadn't yet caught up to the technology boom, and I didn't hesitate to point that out after the first treatment. So she insisted I bring some movies the following week, and once I arrived, she wheeled an old, 1990s-era tube TV and VCR from the back storage area into the chemo room and right in front of my chair. If I wasn't already turning heads of gray, this solidified it. Yet Nurse Kim didn't seem to care. She'd managed to find a key to my heart already, and it was clear: she wasn't letting go.

At first, all I knew about Nurse Kim was that she worked as Dr. Rosen's nurse practitioner and had wig brochures. I also noticed she had short brown hair, small circle-framed glasses, and one of the kindest smiles I'd ever seen. She actually reminded me a lot of my boss, Gayla, from the library, endlessly warm and comforting.

I was glad Nurse Kim sat in on our appointments with Dr. Rosen. Once chemotherapy began, I saw her often. As he and my parents reviewed lab work, Kim asked questions. She wanted to know everything—about my boyfriend, my brother, and my friends at school. My life outside of cancer was important to her too. She'd slowly and swiftly gained so much trust, I began voicing things to Nurse Kim I dared not say to another.

"I should get *something* out of this, like a scholarship!" I teased while hunched in the chair during my third chemo treatment. Already weary and worn down, yearning to return to school, I was dreaming about making it to college and kidding about getting a scholarship for surviving. Lo and behold, Kim searched online and found one: the American Cancer Society's Young Cancer Survivor Scholarship.

"You should apply for this next year!" She beamed as she put printouts into my hand. In her mind, there was no question. I would beat this cancer and go on to college, and I would get this scholarship! It was the first of many times Nurse Kim would show her cards—she loved me. She believed in me. She thought my cancer was going to turn into something good. She didn't have to say it; I just knew.

"Oh Danielle, you look so wonderful. I'm so proud of you."

Nearly every time I saw her, she pumped me up with encouraging words. As chemo took its toll, my hair thinned, my skin became dry, and I got really pale. Yet in Nurse Kim's eyes, I was more and more beautiful. The week I couldn't find my smile to flash back at her, she ran to her office and came back with a gift: a white basket with a medallion saying "Hope" hanging off of it.

"This is my hope basket, but I want you to have it," she said.

I was shocked. I mean, I was far from her *only* patient at the cancer center; the chairs were full every week. But she knew I needed the boost, and I appreciated it. Maybe she could tell I wasn't exactly making friends. Confused looks from both the other patients getting infusions and the caregivers keeping them company were the norm. I assumed they didn't know how to handle a patient my age, and that was why most of them didn't talk to me. A seventeen-year-old cancer patient? Watch out for the attitude. They had no clue.

It did feel lonely at times, but I honestly hardly noticed thanks to Nurse Kim and the others on her team. When I could have gone low, they lifted me high. I didn't slump into the same depression I saw etched onto other patients' faces. They were insistent—I had nothing to look forward to but life. The seasons were changing in agreement.

The trees behind the windowpanes of the infusion room were bare branches when I'd first walked in, but after several months, they were blooming with buds of pink and green. The days were getting warmer. The grass was growing greener. Drizzles of rain served as an announcement for spring. I assumed the changing of seasons meant something different to each patient, but for me it meant one very unique thing. It was a moment I'd been waiting for even before I'd heard the words "You have cancer." Springtime brought the prom.

I stood in my room facing the mirror, and for the first time in a long time, I truly, joyfully smiled. Makeup highlighted my face, and my red satin dress created small waves each time I shuffled back and forth. I looked like a princess.

I'd spent the entire Saturday getting ready for the dance. I knew if I wanted to stay up and be out past nine o'clock, I needed to "go slow." That morning after waking up, I'd rested on the couch and watched TV. In the early afternoon, I took a hot shower and carefully scrubbed off the sticky tape residue. While it worked well to hold cotton balls against my skin after nurses stuck needles into my veins, it didn't go with an evening gown. I'd also slowly washed and dried my short hair, and I had never felt so thankful it was there. After I started chemotherapy, it had begun thinning, and I cut it pixie-style short so I wouldn't see so much come out in handfuls. Whether it was the special conditioner my grandma, a beautician, encouraged Mom to buy, or the power of my heartfelt prayers, I didn't know. But my hair hadn't *completely* fallen out, just thinned a lot. By the dance, it had grown a little and was long enough to (sort of) curl.

I knew the other girls from school spent their mornings at salons and makeup counters getting fancy updos and professional looks. At one point in my life, I would have felt insecure to not join them, but after only four short months of fighting colon cancer, a lot had changed. I couldn't feel anything but grateful.

A joyful smile arose as I looked into the mirror, and it came from somewhere deep. It was a place that wasn't new, perhaps, but a place that had, over the years, gotten buried. The colonoscopy, surgeries, appointments, and treatments had covered it up the past few months. But the truth was, my joy had been buried even before that. Between hating my body, hiding my parents' secrets, and seeing blood specks in the toilet, my true smile had gone away. Cancer was actually helping me rediscover it.

Had I focused on the days leading up to the prom, I would have struggled to even grin. Dr. Rosen, along with doctors at M. D. Anderson, agreed I needed radiation therapy in addition to chemo. My tumor was considered both colon and rectal cancer, since it sat

> *Between hating my body, hiding my parents' secrets, and seeing blood specks in the toilet, my true smile had gone away. Cancer was actually helping me rediscover it.*

right in the middle where the two parts connected. This meant I added yet another stop on my medical carousel: Dr. Jorge Paradelo, whom I came to adore. He was the happiest, most positive, and most excited doctor of anyone on my team. I genuinely believed he felt thrilled I'd become his patient.

His attitude was appreciated because it helped me transition into yet another doctor's office to face more questioning, invasive pokes, and prods. His visits unfortunately came with frequent rectal exams, which I hated as much as all of them. But I'd learned how to grin and bear it and put my mind on happy things. Finishing treatment. Having no evidence of disease (they actually had an acronym for this: NED). Going back to school as a senior. And having Mike take me to prom. These were happy thoughts and milestones I set that got me through fears that wore on.

Treatment was building and bringing a new level of fatigue, but preparing for one of the most monumental nights of my teenage life kept me energized. One day when I felt well enough, Mom and I visited a special occasions store we saw advertised in the newspaper. It was a sight to behold—glass windows with sparkling gowns gleaming on the inside. It was a much different sight than the plain cinder block walls of hospitals and medical clinics I'd been frequenting. As we stepped inside the store, something felt magical. Dresses of nearly every color hung on circular racks, and there were more beads, sparkles, and shimmers than I'd seen in my entire life.

While the selections felt endless, a bright-red dress quickly popped out to both Mom and me. It was one of the first gowns we saw. It had a few beads near the bust area and a strappy back that added a simple elegance.

"Do you want to try it on?" the store clerk asked.

Even before I pulled back the curtain to show my mom, I knew. "This is the one."

As I stepped out to the three-paneled mirror, everyone in the store could see. I was glowing. The dress had transformed me. I didn't look like a tired teenage cancer patient, but I felt pretty enough to be a queen. Although I saw what I would have once considered flaws—the bump in my chest from the Port-a-Cath and very pale skin since I had to stay away from the sun, I embraced them because they were part of my story. It also didn't hurt that I was wearing a size small.

I changed out of the dress, and Mom paid for it. The weeks that followed were consumed with finding the perfect shoes, earrings, and makeup. The chemo nurses asked for an update each time I went in for a treatment, seeming to be even more excited for the dance than I was.

Life was a balance. I'd get new gear for prom, and then I'd get new gear for chemo, like a continuous (24-7, yes, I took it to bed) infusion pump I nicknamed Chester. The home health nurse informed me that once the prom was over, I'd be wearing the pump all the time so I could get both chemo and radiation. Two very different paths with very different plans seemed to be running on the same timeline. But the prom pathway gave me energy and life. It helped me face all the icky stuff that radiation would soon bring—the tattoos and sunburns on my bottom, the abdominal pain, and the laser beams. It was stuff that would have been hard to handle had I not been distracted by the upcoming event I considered epic, amazing.

It felt like the days leading up to prom unspooled so slowly until the Saturday it actually arrived. When I finally stood at the mirror by late afternoon, I was glad I'd taken the whole day to get ready. Thankful for the ability to slow down and soak it all in, I stood in the mirror and looked at a brave teenager draped in red. I hardly recognized myself. It was true—the sparkles, makeup, and fancy gown were a sight I'd never seen. But more than that, I'd approached the mirror differently this time. Cancer had once again changed me.

For so many years—not months—before cancer, I'd approached the mirror with sadness and disappointment. When I saw my reflection, I had thoughts of criticism and shame. I'd picked on myself for every flaw and imperfection. I couldn't see anything good. Certainly not strength.

But thanks to cancer, gazing at my own reflection brought something new. I actually wasn't embarrassed by what I saw. For once, I thought, *Wow, I look beautiful.*

I was proud simply to be alive, standing tall and well enough to get made up and dressed up. As I stared into my own eyes, my mind flashed back to a not-so-distant memory. It had happened at this very mirror the night before my first surgery.

Our houseful of praying visitors had cleared out, and I faced the vanity mirror once the house went quiet. I'd lifted up my shirt just above the elastic band of my pajama pants and began to trace an invisible line with my finger. Remembering the sketch in Dr. Connor's office,

I tried to picture my abdomen with a scar. I stared at my flat, unblemished stomach and wished I would have appreciated it more.

My midsection had never been good enough for me, nor had my skin tone, hips, and teeth. I'd insisted on getting braces just months before starting my junior year in the hopes I'd at least have a perfect smile. But after four months

But if a body that was still standing after facing what I'd endured wasn't perfect, I wasn't sure what was.

of living with colon cancer as a teenager, all of that had turned around. My body was still far from perfect—at least that was what the magazines would say. But if a body that was still standing after facing what I'd endured wasn't perfect, I wasn't sure what was.

As I soaked in the moment, tears threatened to stream down my face. But I refused to let them, mostly because I didn't want to ruin my dark eye makeup. Fortunately, the doorbell rang, and the long-awaited evening began. I heard the hinges on our front door squeak as my parents welcomed Mike into our house. I puckered my lips one more time, checked my lipstick, and opened my bedroom door to head for the stairs.

In what felt like a grand entrance, I stopped to grab the railing. The last thing any of us needed was for me to fall. Mike stood next to Mom and Dad, and all three of them broke out tooth-filled smiles. This wasn't just my exciting moment. It took all of us to reach this point.

Mike looked so handsome in a tuxedo and home-sewn red vest. Once his mom heard about my red gown, she'd found some fabric to match it. While away at college, Mike dyed his hair, and blond highlights shot through his small curls. They were extra defined for our special evening; I could tell he had even used hair gel.

Although we'd been to homecoming and a few other dances together, I'd never seen Mike look so nice. I absolutely loved that under his sleeves and buttoned-up collar he still wore his FROG bracelet and bottle-cap necklace. As I slowly made it down the stairs, Mike offered me his arm. We didn't care that Mom and Dad were watching us. I wrapped my arms around his neck for a huge hug. We'd made it! It was going to be one of the best nights ever, not because we had romantic plans to sneak off, but because we were finally getting to act our age and just be together.

Mike slipped a beautiful flower corsage with white roses onto my wrist, and I pinned a matching bouton-niere to his lapel. We took a few pictures on the deck before leaving to take more pictures with our friends. Emily helped coordinate a small group, and we met at a friend's house.

"Okay, look this way!"

"Now me!"

It felt awesome, yet surreal, to be standing along a banister with other girls in formal dresses. I'd forgotten what it felt like to be in high school. We said goodbye to our parents after pictures, loaded into a van, and got ready to drive off.

"Do you have the phone?" Dad asked, helping me feel cool for once. He had recently purchased a mobile phone that we kept in the car. None of my other friends had traded pagers for phones yet, but he didn't want me going anywhere without it.

"Yeah, in my purse," I said. It also helped me feel more secure. In case of an emergency, he was one call away.

We drove to a Japanese steakhouse for dinner, where I tried my "seal best" to catch the flying shrimp the cook tossed at me from the grill with my mouth (unsuccessfully). After dinner, we drove to the big pavilion, where everyone else from school was pulling into the parking lot. Getting out of the van, I started to feel a little nervous.

What if I get tired or fall? What if dinner doesn't sit well? What if somebody's here and I get their germs and feel sick? Should I hug people or keep my distance and stay away?

Mike reached over and took my arm, reminding me I wasn't alone. He could tell by the look on my face that I was getting overwhelmed. But with his soft touch, I remembered that no matter what, it was a godsent night. We walked into the room, which was full of twinkling lights and decorations. Girls in long gowns swayed on the dance floor with their dates. Above them, a disco ball hung and spun tiny square lights all across the room as the Backstreet Boys played. It was happening. I couldn't even put words to the feeling.

A lot of people gasped when they saw me, shocked I'd made it to prom. I talked to a few friends I'd missed since leaving school, but for most of the night, I danced with Mike. On the fast songs, I'd take a break and sit. On the slow songs, I'd take Mike's hand as he escorted me to the dance floor. He'd pull me in close, I'd rest my hands on his neck, and we'd shuffle our feet from side to side.

We made it. I was alive. We were together. It was a dream. I was careful to not rush the scene. We both knew that eventually, our fairy-tale moment would pass. We'd get back into the car, and he'd drive me home. In a few days, Mike would return to school to finish his classes. Dad would start driving me to radiation oncology, calling them buggy rides, for thirty days. The twinkling lights above us would come down. The slow-dance music would eventually cease. We were living inside our own Cinderella story; the fairy-tale carriage would return to a humble pumpkin.

But in our moment, we didn't think about any of that. As two teenagers in love, we clung to each other. Without a care in the world, unaware of anyone else in the room, I rested my cheek against his shoulder as we ever so gently swayed.

15

Dear Diary

June 22, 2001

I am not a diary writer. But I've finally listened to the people around me and decided to keep a journal. I know that when I'm sixty years old, I will be mad at myself if I don't start writing down my cancer journey. I wrote letters to Mike all last school year before he moved home, but this is different. These entries are just for me.

I'm going to give a little history so I know where I am in my life. In January, I was diagnosed with colon cancer. I've undergone three surgeries so far and have completed around thirteen weeks of cancer treatment. I have six weeks to go. The first bit of chemo made me pretty sick, but I was still able to do some things with my friends off and on. During the beginning of radiation, I was feeling pretty good, but toward the end was not fun. I was on a very strict diet—not even able to eat ketchup! I would not go out of the house much because I was pretty tired, and I wasn't sure I could be away from a bathroom for that long. This week has been much better. My social calendar does not revolve around my bathroom habits. I used to be pretty embarrassed about using the restroom, but not anymore. God really took care of that paranoia. Chemo starts up again next Tuesday. I'm not excited, but I'm looking forward to finishing treatment and beginning my senior year. I missed the last part of my junior year, at least the going to school part. I was not up to daily school life, so I did my classes at home. At first I didn't mind not going to school, but toward the end, I really missed my friends. But senior year is going to be very fun—I can feel it. It has to be!

Twenty Pounds Down

June 23, 2001

I usually write about how I want to lose weight, but not really this time. I've lost around 20 lbs. so far from the treatments. I'm weighing around 128 right now. When I get well, I want to start working out and tone my body. I'm thin but not toned. I haven't lost my hair (it's a miracle!), but I did cut it shorter just in case. I'm very white this summer—but the sun burns my skin quickly due to the chemo. But that's okay—I'm just learning how to be thankful for everything—friends, family, and being alive. And for the Royals baseball game. It should be very fun—it's Buck Night and Fireworks Friday! :)

Soft Taco Supreme Date Night

June 24, 2001

We didn't end up going to the Royals game because they sold out, but Mike and I decided that since we were mainly going for the $1 hotdogs, we would go to Taco Bell instead and eat cheap. I've had a big craving for Soft Taco Supremes, so it was good. Then we went miniature golfing and star gazing. His convertible comes in handy. We don't "go out" like normal couples on dates very often. It's been fun.

Grown Apart

July 7, 2001

As I am nearing the end of my treatment, I realize that I've basically grown apart from everyone except my family and Mike. But I realize that and am working on it. Em and I really want a good, close relationship. Last night I made Mike really upset, and he said it seems like he's always saying sorry—and he's right. Then it hit me that I am the one who needed to do the apologizing. I think that's why we've been in little tiffs a lot. I've been in them with my brother too. Since I've been sick, I've been looked after and catered to—not needing to worry if I was in the wrong. But last night I said sorry, and it felt good.

What Happened to the "Old Danielle"?

July 23, 2001

School starts in less than a month. I guess you could say I'm ready, since I've been dreaming about school starting up again at night. So far I've dreamed that I get a special "go to the bathroom anytime" pass and that I'm never counted tardy to a class. Good luck on that one! Mom and I went shoe shopping yesterday. On the way to the store, we had a good talk. It was kind of an upsetting subject, but I felt good about it because I actually said what I was thinking. I don't really have a side to her and Dad's fighting—I'm beginning to see both sides more and more. Now as I'm older, have gone through a rough trial, and have a good relationship of my own, I see the situation a little differently in some ways. I guess now instead of focusing on how much it's affecting and hurting me, I recognize the problem and take note of it so hopefully I don't mirror it.

Lately I've been getting a lot of "What happened to the old Danielle?" The one who was happy and so full of faith and life all the time? I feel bad because I've changed and really am trying to get back to that, but it's hard. I've had to really use up all the faith I have—unlike many adults today. I'm not showing overjoy all the time right now because my cup is not running over—it's getting filled up constantly, being super careful it doesn't get any cracks and break. I have faith it will get filled back up and overflow again.

LAST DAY OF CHEMO!
July 24, 2001

I am finished with treatment! That's a surprise! I saw Dr. Rosen today, and he sees no immediate reason for me to continue. Praise the Lord! So today has been a celebration. Mom and Dad took me to Eskew's Jewelry store and had me pick out a keepsake for this day. I chose a really nice watch with crystals all around its face. It's very special to me. On the back is engraved "Survivor" and the date. It's neat! Mike brought me some big sunflowers. Tonight we ate at Gojo on the Plaza. It was a super good day.

I'M NOT THE ONLY ONE FIGHTING CANCER
July 31, 2001

I'm at youth camp. I've been praying for God to use my cancer for his glory. Well, tonight I got to talk to a girl whose mom had a brain tumor, and she has been upset and angry, turning to other things. Tonight I shared that you can't let cancer beat you—or it will. I encouraged her to be there for her mom, as the fear of recurrence (it coming back) is real. God has been showing me that cancer is not my world anymore. Not everything can revolve around it. While I will never forget any of the experiences, I cannot constantly use my sickness as an excuse as I rebuild.

I have fought the good fight. I have finished the race,
I have kept the faith (2 Timothy 4:7).

DANIELLE RIPLEY-BURGESS

WHAT KIND OF SONG

Everyone thought, they thought you were super woman.
From the surface, you couldn't be brought down.
Trying so hard to save lives we didn't see it coming.
All the talk was warning signs that it would be around.

Now that it's here we feel the world turn.
Now that it's here we all start to yearn.
The shadow of death is so frightening.
We can't help but start from wondering . . .

What kind of song will come out of this?
Where's the good in such a situation?
Asking why is so hard to resist.
God give us strength as we wait in such expectation.

Everyone thought, they thought it had to be bad,
Where is room for rejoicing?
I wanna cry, I wanna weep, I wanna be sad.
But I've seen God's work and I've seen God's hand.
He's here moving as the world turns.
He's at work while we yearn.
The shadow of death is so frightening,
We can't help but start from wondering.
—Michael Burgess, 2001

16

New Beginnings

"**D**ID YOU GUYS HEAR WHAT happened this morning in New York City with the Twin Towers?"

I looked up at my classmate, who stood on the other side of the bench in the girls' locker room combing her blond hair. Like mine, it was matted and sticky with sweat from our workout. Our cheeks were pink, and we were rushing to get changed. Since the autumn mornings were chilly but bearable, our PE teacher had been taking us on cross-country-like runs through tree-lined dirt paths near the high school.

Although I could have easily asked to skip out on the running, I was more determined than ever to keep up. I'd never been a runner, and I hadn't played sports since I'd quit volleyball, but now as a cancer survivor, I had a new motivation. I felt unstoppable. I courageously rode roller coasters when I went to the amusement park with Mike's family. I jumped off diving boards in a swimming suit and didn't care who watched. And I challenged myself in PE. If I was still alive, I was going to go for it. I would no longer be a shy girl holding back.

The other girls in the locker room didn't respond to our concerned classmate, and I felt relieved. I wasn't the only one who hadn't a clue what was happening in New York City. Shrugging it off, I wasn't too concerned. We lived in the middle of America, right in the heart of the United States, and what happened on the coasts, including NYC, rarely affected us (or so I thought). I hadn't a clue what had happened at the World Trade Center inside the Twin Towers. Plus, I'd been outside running for the past half hour, and my mind was focused on getting my armpit sweat to dry, not national news.

The bell rang, and I tossed my damp gym clothes into my locker before slipping on my backpack and heading for my next class. I was grateful for everything—to be back walking the halls at school. To be strong enough to a lug a heavy backpack. I was glad my hair was growing longer. I was even grateful, oddly, for the ability to be around germs again. I wasn't surrounded by white-haired cancer patients anymore, but instead, everywhere I looked, there were people my age. I never realized how much I missed that until it was gone.

I was especially excited about new friends Emily and I were hanging out with: Leah, a friend I'd known since fourth-grade volleyball; Joy, a new student our senior year; and Adam. Although we'd been friends at school for a long time, we began getting together outside of it. Adam and Mike even started a band with a couple of brothers and filled our nights and weekends with practices and local shows.

Glad to have him living closer again, I was psyched Mike had enrolled in a different college to pursue his teaching degree. He wanted to be with me as much as possible, and I didn't argue. It felt like, already, he loved me unconditionally, and I felt the same way. Although young, we'd lived through so much already. I hoped we'd be in each other's lives, somehow, forever.

On my way to the next class, personal finance, I didn't rush through the halls, but I walked fast enough to avoid being tardy. The football coach taught the class, and his teaching style differed from other classroom teachers. He gave very little homework and tests. He spent the hour lecturing to make things like checks, credit cards, and investments understandable. When he taught about big expenditures and the idea of debt, I realized cancer may have actually *cost* my parents money. Mom and Dad hadn't mentioned it, but I began to wonder what kind of price tag had just been put on my life. Did I now have a million-dollar rear end? I didn't know the actual amounts, but I figured cancer drugs and surgeries weren't cheap.

From the second I walked into Coach's classroom, I knew something was off. The rarely-used TV was on with nearly every eyeball glued to it. Sliding into my seat, I watched as big, gray puffs of smoke surrounded two tall gray buildings—the Twin Towers, I gathered. The World Trade Center was falling down.

The room was quiet, both before and after the bell. What we watched looked like a history movie, except we weren't in history class. The news coverage flipped to the Pentagon. Clearly something was wrong, but before I understood, Coach turned the TV off.

"Okay, ladies and gentlemen, let's try to focus today."

We didn't talk about what we'd just witnessed, nor did Coach attempt to explain.

An hour later, once the bell dismissed us, the halls were buzzing with gossip.

"Did you see the buildings fall? Who do you think did it? What happened?"

We'd not witnessed anything like it. Our generation, the millennials, as people would call us, knew of a world full of peace. The only other image I could recall seeing that looked even remotely similar to the collapsing building had come from the Oklahoma City bombing when I was much younger. *This* seemed even worse and more severe. It had never occurred to me, nor the others in the hallways, that someone from outside the US could attack our country.

As the day turned to afternoon and evening, fragmented pieces came slowly together. After school, I flipped on our TV at home and learned the buildings had fallen because of an attack. From channel to channel, it was the only topic being discussed. Pictures of ash-covered New Yorkers running down the street in high heels. Jumpers escaping the fires atop the tall buildings. Firemen rushing into the flames. It was pure horror. Along with the rest of the world, I watched in disbelief.

Terrorists had flown airplanes into important buildings. A lot of people had just died. I instantly felt the gravity and the loss of those who were suffering. Cancer had given me a unique ability to empathize.

In the week following the Tuesday attack, the *Kansas City Star* delivered a special issue to each home containing a newsprint version of the American flag folded inside. Within minutes of the paper hitting our driveways, we taped the flag to our front doors. As I drove through our neighborhood, I'd see flag after flag. It was somber and sad, yet incredibly unifying. What had once divided neighbors was suddenly gone. From the house with the yappy dog to the house with the year-round Christmas lights, everyone was suddenly equal. Our little annoyances didn't matter anymore.

I instantly felt the gravity and the loss of those who were suffering. Cancer had given me a unique ability to empathize.

In addition to the flags, cities all across the country held rallies, including our suburban town. We all bought T-shirts promising to "Never Forget" and gathered on our high school football field to salute the flag, honor first responders, and pay tribute to those who lost their lives in New York City, an area which suddenly didn't seem *so* far away. The attacks were terrifying and horrific, and we were all scared. Yet they were also bringing our community, and the nation at large, together. We were Americans. We were neighbors.

It was an interestingly odd time to be taking everything in. Not only was I unsure about how to step out of high school and into a world under a threat of terror, but I was doing it as someone who'd just survived my own personal attack, cancer. Watching my neighbors cope with the scrolling headlines following 9/11 gave me language and understanding for what I'd recently lived through. I could relate to the fears. *Is it going to strike again? Where did it come from? Where did I go wrong?* Yet I also found a determined optimism. *I will stand firm. I will never forget. I will survive.*

Although our country's mood felt heavy following the terrorist attacks and subsequent war, things in my life were actually looking up. It didn't take me long to rejoin my teenage life, and the daily focus became school, youth group, and, of course, Mike. Unlike most of my classmates, I didn't suffer from "senioritis" and daydream about graduation. I'd wanted nothing more than to get back *into* the school. I wasn't in a hurry to get out. Yet as graduation neared, I did find myself feeling excited not only to walk across a stage wearing a cap and gown, but to attend the formal dances. Mike and I attended my senior homecoming dance in fall, and after Christmas there were only two more left: winter formal, or court-warming, and senior prom.

As school tradition held, a few weeks before each formal dance, the classes nominated and voted on one guy and girl to represent them as part of a royal court. The senior class chose four guys and four girls to be on the court, and a few weeks before the dance, they voted on the dance's king and queen. Ever since my fresh-man-year homecoming dance, I'd participated by voting for the athletes, cheerleaders, dancers, and theater leads nominated to represent us. Although I wasn't into popularity contests, I enjoyed our formal dance traditions. The nominees were typically those who sat far away from my lunch table, but it was still fun to join in. "I nominated you!" I was shocked—total disbelief—when a friend mentioned that she had nominated me for courtwarming queen.

"Who, me?" I gasped, flattered at the thought while laughing off the possibility. There was no way someone like me would ever get voted into the royal court, cancer survivor or not. But a few weeks later, I wasn't laughing anymore.

"Danielle Ripley!"

My name was being called not by a nurse wanting me to follow her, but by the school secretary. Over the loudspeaker, her voice echoed throughout the locker-lined halls as she rattled off the top four senior girls nominated for the courtwarming royal court. It had to be a mistake—me? Out of a class of nearly four hundred students, I was up for *queen*? In the three years prior, I'd not been nominated to represent our class once. My name had *never* come up. As the news soaked in, I began to wonder if my classmates had noticed my absence all along. I gladly accepted the nomination.

Royal court came with several fun traditions. For starters, I returned to the photography studio I'd visited a year prior, but this time, I wasn't getting photographed because of a looming threat of hair loss. As a treat to us seniors, the school requested our portraits. I smiled wide at the sound of the flash, now unphased by my shorter hair and braces. Trying to hide my emotion, I smiled wide. I didn't want to cry in front of my classmates or the adults, nor was I open to talking about the big feelings rising up inside. Yet behind the smile and twinkling eyes was a deep appreciation. I'd returned to the same photo backdrop not only alive, but as a potential queen.

"I doubt I'll win," I told several friends, guarding myself against the disappointment I expected to follow. Truly, I felt honored to be nominated, and a little dumbfounded. Our class had nominated several queen candidates whom I happened to be friends with. I felt most of them had a better shot at winning, yet I couldn't help but imagine sometimes. *What would a crown on my head really feel like?* The thought felt unbelievable and strange.

"Oh, I think you've got this. You can win it!" friends and family said, convinced I could rack in the most votes. But I didn't believe it could happen, even up to the minute when I saw the local newspaper's front-page headline.

"BELIEVE IT OR NOT, RIPLEY'S THE QUEEN!"

During halftime of the Friday night varsity basketball game, the whirlwind began. A loud buzzer took the game into halftime, and eventually the bouncing basketballs stopped. The buttery smell of freshly popped popcorn wafted in from the concession stand as teachers, reporters, and photographers huddled in the middle of the court to indicate, "It's showtime!" The crowd in the bleachers hushed as the squeal from a scratchy microphone got everyone's attention.

The freshman guy and girl at the front of the line each took their parents' arms and walked slowly onto the court as their names were announced. It felt like a wedding reception grand entrance, except there was no groom, bride, or pastel gowns. The guys were in suits, and the girls wore A-line pencil skirts with matching jackets. Our lips were red, and our hair was curled. We looked at once pretty and conservative.

"Danielle Ripley and her father."

Dad and I followed the path the others walked and found our place along the semicircle forming on the court. Once we made it to where the organizers asked us to stop, I looked up into the crowd. There weren't many open seats; it was nearly standing room only. At one point, I would have wanted to melt into a puddle with so many eyes on me, but I'd changed. I stood tall, chin up, and smiled. Classmates were smiling, waving. It was incredibly empowering—and healing. Maybe they cared after all.

Once all the senior candidates and their parent escorts made their way to the semicircle, a wave of "Shh-hhhhhhhhh" got everyone to quiet down. We all knew what was coming next. I wondered if anyone could hear my heart nearly beating out of my chest.

"And the 2002 Courtwarming Queen is . . ."

I held my breath, gripped Dad's arm even tighter, and looked down at my knocking knees.

"Danielle *Rip*ley!"

The crowd erupted, as did a volcano of joy inside my heart. Flashes from the photographer clicked off as the previous year's queen placed a crown atop my head and a bouquet of red roses into my arms. I imagined anyone in the crowd who knew my story might have been tearing up. I was holding them back myself. I couldn't wipe the awestruck grin off my face as I took the arm of my friend

Greg, who'd been voted king. We smiled for the photographer and waved to the crowd. I couldn't believe it. I was an official queen.

Thumping, bouncing basketballs and a buzzer meant the basketball game was back on, so I walked to the foyer, where Mom, Andy, and Mike met me. Mom beamed with pride. Mike grabbed me for a hug. He was feeling a similar disbelief.

How is this possible? How is it happening?

Just one year prior, I'd been told I'd had cancer and found myself in the fight of my life. Now I was carrying a bouquet of roses with a crown on my head, receiving congratulations from people I both did and didn't know.

Me—the queen. It was surreal. The local newspaper came out a few days later to do a story not only about the courtwarming queen, but the cancer journey that (I assumed) had led up to the crown. I appreciated their tongue-in-cheek headline. They were right—unbelievable. A few months later, TV stations caught wind of my story and came to the house to do stories too. The seventeen-year-old from the suburbs who had beaten colon cancer was suddenly hot news.

I wanted to be honest in case anyone saw blood in the toilet too. Maybe they wouldn't have to get cancer.

Answering the reporter's questions also felt surreal because for the first time, I was speaking publicly, vulnerably, about my body and cancer. When asked about symptoms, I said I'd felt embarrassed about my body and hid that I saw blood in the stool. I even used the word *hemorrhoids*. I couldn't believe I was telling a reporter—on the record—about what I'd once hidden from everyone! I wanted to be honest in case anyone saw blood in the toilet too. Maybe they wouldn't have to get cancer.

When several articles and stories came out, they covered it all—including my high school graduation, beating cancer, and future college plans. I'd felt the still, small voice lead me to a university closer to home in central Missouri with a globally recognized public relations program. I'd even received a scholarship from the American Cancer Society—the one Nurse Kim found—to help pay for some of the costs.

The media had covered the story of my life to a tee. Except for one missing part, which I intentionally left out. I didn't mention what was happening with Mom and Dad and how, unlike my health, my family wasn't going to make it.

I knew fighting was a part of all relationships, especially as Mike and I started dating. Although we didn't fight much, we did have our moments, especially when the future came up. Mike wanted to be a rock star, yet I was already wanting to talk about settling down.

"You're going to leave me to go on tour!" I'd sulk.

"No, I'm not," he'd insist in a shaky-voiced reply. He wanted both—was that possible? I wanted him to accomplish his big dreams too (even if that did mean leaving town). When his band eventually broke up in college, I hoped it wasn't my fault. Give and take, ebb and flow, I knew that relationships took work. I could tell that whatever was happening between Mom and Dad was not only unhealthy, but eventually beyond repair.

For years, I'd prayed about their discussions and hoped Mom and Dad would get along. Sometimes it felt like answers. The fighting stopped. Mom and Dad went on a date. At one point, they even recarpeted the house, put in new landscaping, and bought new furniture.

It's working! Thank you, God!

But (kind of like my no-red-foods diet, come to think of it) nothing stuck, and the tension returned. After a while, it never left. It didn't matter if we were at a school assembly, where I was receiving a scholarship, or my graduation ceremony, where I tossed my cap into the air. The tension was ever present. It followed us into follow-up appointments with doctors and into Emily's and my dorm room as we carried in our futon and mini fridge during move-in day. Both big and small moments brought a chronic fear that something between Mom and Dad would explode—or implode. And a few weeks following an awfully tense, uncomfortable winter break during my first year of college, I got the long-awaited call.

"Mom moved out . . ."

It was Andy. I'd just been home for Christmas, and we had a feeling their marriage was worse than ever and could be ending soon. We'd been right. I didn't have much to say in response, not to Andy nor to Mom and Dad, who each drove to see me and make their case over dinner. Although I was glad to be out of the house and at out, I felt bad for Andy. He was one semester away from graduating high school. Why would this be happening during his senior year? Hadn't his sister getting cancer during his sophomore year and his own health challenges been enough? Now this? I wished I could make it better.

A roller coaster of grief soon kicked in as I went from feeling relieved, angry, sad, and grateful throughout the course of a day. Oftentimes, I'd sit on the futon with Mike's arm around me in disbelief. Barely seventeen, I'd fought for my life and beaten cancer. Now I was barely nineteen, and my parents were splitting. It didn't seem fair, especially when I compared myself to the students on campus who appeared to have zero worries other than ordering Chinese takeout and cramming for tests.

"Lord, I'm not sure I can handle any more," I'd pray quietly as I'd walk between tall campus buildings to get to and from class. My heart ached all the time. Fortunately, unlike high school, I realized that despite yet another crisis, my friends and several family members weren't ignoring or excluding me. In a welcome turn of events, several actually dared to come in close to make sure I knew they cared.

Shortly after college classes began, Grandma Rose Mary mailed me a handwritten letter each week filling me in on life at her farm and the weather. Emily and I also stayed really close, and she was a great roommate— super clean! Seeing her each day reminded me of my thirteenth birthday and waking up to read Job. She carried a reminder that God wasn't far away—He would help me get through anything. Several other friends who lived on our hall often came by to play games or watch

TV, and Leah from high school hung out with us too. It was all a welcome distraction.

But few others made me feel more loved than a girl named Amber who hung out in our dorm. I instantly liked her. Once, while eating dinner at a greasy Mexican joint, things clicked further—it felt like we'd been friends forever. Our upbringings couldn't have been more different other than the fact our parents made sure we grew up in Christian homes. She was from a rural town with fewer than three thousand people, and I was from one of the biggest suburbs in the state, touting a population just shy of one hundred thousand. I'd never even heard of jumping hay, moving cattle, and growing alfalfa until I met her, which was part of her family's everyday life. She played softball and loved to accessorize. I hadn't done sports for years and barely remembered to wear earrings. Despite being night-and-day different, we easily and instantly got along.

Amber and I often took walks around campus, and I found it funny she insisted on wearing flip-flops, even if it was snowing outside. On weekends, we'd drive to shop at the outlets or peruse old antique stores. She and Mike became fast friends, too, and we all joined an intramural volleyball team. In the midst of my family falling apart, Amber invited me to hers. Weekend hangouts occasionally became road trips to her childhood home, where both Mike and I got a dose of the country. The open fields and dirt roads became healing, far away from the chaos back home. The countryside brought respite with its soothing sights and sounds, which became coupled with helpful books and note cards from Aunt Deb.

Of all my relatives, she'd always been *the* birthday card sender, never missing a date (And usually the card would arrive right on time—I had no idea how she did that!) But once my parents split, Aunt Deb rushed in even closer—and quickly. Perhaps she knew my faith was shaken; my church-going family foundation had just been destroyed. Late-night phone calls and frequent care packages in the mail from her reminded me that God had a big plan for my life. Sometimes she sent encouraging books. Other times, verses written on note cards to stick to my dorm room walls. She invited me to Christian women's conferences and recommended Bible studies. While tempted to turn from faith, thanks to my support system, I pressed on. I couldn't see it right away, but I wanted to believe the encouragement. God had good plans in store for me.

How could any good could come from my parents' divorce? Unlike cancer, it would take time to see. But in the present, despite everything else collapsing, there was still one shiny part of my life—Mike.

He'd seen it happening; Mike was around our house so much, my parents eventually stopped hiding their disputes from him. He'd heard the bickering. Picked up on the secrets. Yet he'd stayed.

Am I now damaged goods? I feared. Yet in his eyes, no way.

I'd overheard concerns from parents when their adult kids showed interest in dating someone from a broken home. Compared to Mike's family, which appeared to be the epitome of perfect and happy, mine was a wreck. His parents and sister were involved in Christian organizations doing youth ministry. They were a model family, what I'd hoped and prayed ours could be. Between my cancer and now this, who would want to *be* with me?

But Mike did, and he seemed unfazed by all of it—the cancer, the divorce. He didn't distance himself, but instead, he came closer. He'd stop by to see me every morning in my dorm room and return in the evening once he finished classes. He stood up for me, unshakably, if I got treated unfairly. When the tears broke loose, he dabbed them. When I needed someone to hold me, he volunteered. He always made sure I had a safe place to be, whether it was his house, his car, or in his arms. He also made sure we had fun together, like searching for treasures at CD stores or taking ballroom dancing classes.

During a time in which nobody would have blamed me for never wanting a long-term relationship, myself included, Mike kept romancing my heart. While many of my friends also would have understood if I declared, "I am *never* getting married," I actually wanted nothing more.

17

True Love

I FELL FAST.

After only a few weeks into dating, I sensed Mike was "the one." He had to be. I knew that deep down, he sensed I was the one for him too, although maybe not as fast.

7-31-01

Dear Danielle,

This morning I got up and started reading an article in *Readers Digest*, "Marriage in America: The Secrets That We Keep." There's a story in it about a wife who got breast cancer. The husband says, "I think when your marriage is strong, the tough times only make it stronger. Every time you've shared a problem with another person, you cut the load in half." I know we aren't married, but I thought the quote and article were cool. I

wouldn't have even read it if it weren't for you.
(That's a good thing.)
—Michael

At ages seventeen and twenty, we had marriage on
the mind, although we would have denied it if anyone
asked. But I couldn't imagine anyone ever knowing me
so well, or loving me as deeply, as Mike. He felt the same
way. Mike knew what every wrinkle line on my face
meant and every pause in my voice. Although I wouldn't
tell my girlfriends when "that time of the month" came,
for some reason, I told Mike. He celebrated when I went
poop. I knew his daily bathroom schedule too. We had
fun together—whether we were sitting on the couch
watching sitcoms and eating Cheez-Its or watching local
bands perform. Plus, getting closer to him was safe. We
shared a mutual commitment.

I'd never forgotten what I noticed on the day I met
him. He wore a ball-chained silver necklace with an
oversized silver bottle cap. As we became friends, I was
curious what it meant and why he didn't leave home
without it.

"What's that bottle cap?"

It was an ordinary day, and I was asking my friend
an ordinary question. An awkward silence followed as he
flipped it around so I could see the engraving.

True Love Waits.

Intense feelings of respect and awe filled my chest.
He didn't need to explain it—I knew. I'd first heard about
True Love Waits at youth group a few years after one of
Mom's and my girl talks, the one where she explained

babies get made by sex and that once girls start periods, they can get pregnant. Mom said God made sex for married people, which was fine by me. I was still unable to say the word period without my face turning bright red. Sex had become one of the grossest parts of the whole conversation about growing up and puberty. I wanted nothing to do with it and planned to stay far away, maybe forever.

Although I'd matured since our initial talk in elementary school, I still wasn't ready or comfortable with the True Love Waits teenage campaign (especially since we were discussing it at church!). But I sat through the lessons and, although I stayed quiet, paid close attention.

"Obeying God's commandments is a way to show your love for Him, including sexual purity," the lesson began. I couldn't argue with them, except for the parts where they referred to sex as "beautiful." Yuck. Although I was older and some of my friends seemed curious about it, I wasn't interested at all. I'd never forgotten the shame of seeing an explicit website in fourth grade. I liked the idea of guarding myself under a godly excuse.

During one of the lessons, one of the older girls was brave enough to ask a question I dared not voice. "What if someone doesn't wait until they're married?"

I held my breath to hear our teacher's response. Since it sounded like purity was such a big deal, I was expecting to hear horrible things about God's punishment. But instead, our teachers brought up grace. And then they changed the subject. We didn't talk about True Love Waits at youth group anymore. And while the subject came and went at church, the Christian magazine for

Christian girls I got each month kept talking about it. Throughout its pages were girls a little older than me with stories about their promises to "wait" by signing a pledge. There were national gatherings, weekend conferences, and all kinds of shirts and rings for sale. As I flipped through the products with *True Love Waits*, a silver engraved ring caught my eye. A few days later, it kept coming to mind.

"Mom, I want this for my birthday."

In the same way I'd once circled toys in the Sears holiday catalog, I dropped the magazine into her lap folded to the page with the circled ring. I didn't explain why I wanted it, and she didn't ask. I hadn't talked about sex with her since she first explained it. But after a lot of thinking, reading, and praying on my own, I wanted to sign the pledge and make the promise. To myself. To my future husband. To my future kids. And to God. The ring would remind me.

My parents were often quick to fulfill my wish lists, and they bought me the ring. I acted surprised when I opened it and slipped it on. In the privacy of my bedroom later that night, I took out the green pledge card that came with the ring and signed my name at the bottom. I didn't rush out and show them. In fact, I didn't tell anybody. I tucked the card away into one of my journals. It was ultimately between me and God.

As I got older and started to occasionally date guys, I began to understand the big promise I'd made. It was hard to stop at kissing. I wondered if anyone would date me knowing they wouldn't get more. Slowly, it also became obvious that not all my friends, even those in the youth group, felt the same way about purity. The moment I realized Mike's necklace matched the ring on my finger, I felt relieved.

"Wow. I'm not the only one."

He too had stumbled across the campaign and made a private decision to wait; he even bought the necklace for himself. As we went from just friends to a couple, a lot of things changed. But the purity pledges we individually made to God and ourselves stayed the same. As the years went on and our relationship grew more serious, we realized the promises on our cards were for each other. No matter how tempted we felt, we stuck to them.

"Really? You two are still together?"

I smiled awkwardly, not because of what was said but at the odd position of my feet as my gynecologist blurted it out. With my heels resting in two stirrups and a hopeless hospital gown failing miserably at offering even the slightest bit of modesty, I laughed uncomfortably. Although seeing women in this position was what the doctor and her nurses were used to all day long, it was my first time sitting in such a humiliating chair and having someone perform "a lady exam." It was almost as awful as the rectal exams, but she was a woman, and I did have a choice to be there. I'd been highly encouraged to begin seeing her after my cancer treatments finished. I assumed this was partly because of my cancer risk and partly because everyone *assumed* Mike and I were sleeping together.

"How's your boyfriend?" she asked, I assumed, to be nice.

I was pleased she remembered him, but then again I imagined I was a pretty memorable case. I'd met Dr. Hunter just before radiation began. Dr. Paradelo didn't like the idea of radiating my pelvis without any type of fertility or hormone preservation. We didn't have time to preserve any eggs, but Dr. Hunter performed a surgery that suspended my ovaries (away from radiation targets) in an effort to extend their lifetime. I thought Dr. Hunter was a nice enough lady, but a little firmer and more direct than my other docs. She explained things in a way that made it clear that as she talked, a lot of information ran through her head. But unlike everyone else on my medical carousel, she was a she. I instantly felt more comfortable around a female ob-gyn. And I appreciated that she took an interest in my personal life.

"He's good!" I grinned. "We're going to attend the same college when I graduate!"

Dr. Hunter stopped everything, as did her nurse Donna, whom I adored. With hands on her hips, Dr. Hunter gave me a serious look. "You are still together?" She seemed surprised.

"Yep, we are . . . it's been one and a half years."

Standing still, she stopped to look me right in the eyes. "I meet a lot of women with cancer in this office every day, and a lot of their husbands leave them. If your boyfriend has stuck with you through all this so far, I'd say marry him."

I laughed uncomfortably again, yet this time it wasn't because of my stirruped feet. I loved it when people encouraged my relationship with Mike, but I was nowhere near being ready for marriage. That wasn't to say I hadn't thought about it, especially since we had faced cancer together. Each weekend that Mike drove up to see me, or during the scary moments when he'd hold my hand, I'd thought, *I could marry this guy*. It was just nice, yet surprising, to hear someone else say it—especially since I was only eighteen.

"Ha-ha, okay." I responded quickly, unsure of what else to do or say. But I tucked away Dr. Hunter's advice and never forgot it, even if it looked as if I did. Over the next couple of years, Mike and I were still nearly inseparable outside of a couple more times we put our relationship on pause. I'd dated him since I was sixteen years old. I was the second official girlfriend he'd ever had. All we knew was each other. Sometimes that was great, and other times scary. In a moment, we'd convince ourselves we'd be better off as just friends. But hours, or sometimes a day or two later, we'd realize we were idiots and get back together again. The day I started college, we were back together for good. And three years after that day, on Friday evening following my final exams, we made it official.

"Will you marry me?"

Mike's hands were shaking as he held a white ring box and balanced himself on one knee. A dark sky dotted with bright stars floated above us, and the song "Godsend" was playing on the car stereo. It was an unexpected ending to a perfect evening, although I had a hunch something was up. Mike had asked to take me on a date to the Plaza and even lined up a carriage ride. We'd been talking about getting married, especially since he'd grad-uated college and was about to start working. But I still had years of college left to finish, and I doubted Dad would give Mike his blessing. I'd guessed wrong. Dad said okay as long as Mike promised to work and ensure I always had health insurance. Dad also insisted I graduate college. The love of my life, the man who'd already been with me through sickness and in health, had my dad's blessing and was asking me to be his wife. There was only one reply.

"Yes!"

I planned our wedding for an entire year. From the Friday evening on May 7 that we got engaged to Sat-urday, May 7, one year later, I was a fiancée, a blushing bride. Although I was young, barely twenty-one years old, Mike and I had dated for five years, and many of our wedding guests didn't only say "Congratulations!" but "Finally!" It felt like "finally" to us too.

Just minutes after we got engaged, I became a stu-dent of bridal magazines. Several were waiting for me in the trunk of Mike's car after he proposed, a sign of his confidence in my answer. I quickly knew I wanted a sim-ple but elegant wedding, and something bright. All our parents were generous and offered to chip in and help pay for the wedding, yet they let me decide all the details.

Our colors were easy to choose—green (my favorite) and blue (his). We secured the sanctuary in our home-town church. I liked the traditional feel not only because

I'd grown up in church but also because everything else about my life felt so untraditional. I wanted iconic—and normal. A different venue across town hosted our reception so we could serve a big meal, play loud music, and dance.

For so many years, life was full of back-to-back hard things. But once I got engaged, life started to turn around. Or maybe I was determined to see it that way, whether or not it *was* any different. A wedding to plan gave me something to look forward to, a year full of starry-eyed hope. Just like my junior prom helped get me through chemotherapy, planning a wedding helped me accept what I could not change or control.

Instead of focusing on what went wrong in life, I saw what was right. My focus was turned to wedding dress shopping and finding a beautiful white gown. I taste-tested wedding cakes—my favorite food. My childhood bedroom got packed up so I could move into a duplex with Mike. When *both* of my parents requested to bring "plus-ones," I was surprised but obliged (and later on, very glad they'd brought their dates, since they went on to remarry them). From the showers my bridesmaids threw to the programs, slideshows, and photography, I was hoping for a perfect day. I'd survived a lot to experience it.

Our guest list was large, and we struggled cutting it down. Not only did we share many friends and family, but we also had a host of doctors and nurses to invite. They'd done so much to keep me alive, I wanted them to witness their impact. It warmed my heart when their RSVPs floated in. It also meant a lot to have so many special people involved in our wedding.

Kristi gladly accepted my request and became my matron of honor. Emily; Amber; and Mike's sister, Laura, also said yes to becoming bridesmaids. Mike asked his best friends from high school, George and Darren, to stand next to him, along with a fellow guitarist, Nick, and my brother, Andy. We wanted to avoid a huge wedding party on the stage, but we also wanted to honor several other friends—especially longtime buds like Courtney and Leah, and Jordan from youth group. The influence of Camp Shamineau never faded. Nick, my youth minister, performed the ceremony, and Leslie led their two kids down the aisle as our flower girl and ring bearer. It was a beautiful reunion full of so many people we loved and adored.

"I don't know of many other couples who've been through what you've been through," Nick said, and he challenged us before we said our vows. "You'll be a big help to other couples who, in the future, face some of the hard things you've already had to face."

Staring into each other's eyes, we were ready for the opportunity. There was nothing I wanted more than to slip a ring on his finger and say "I do."

So I did.

"That was one of the most beautiful ceremonies I've ever seen," Mirella insisted as she left the church. And she wasn't talking about the colorful spring flower bouquets, the green bells of Ireland hanging in our pew decorations, or the original song our friend Daren performed, one that Mike had written me for our wedding day. In planning the ceremony, Mike and I had prayed through every part, from the Bible verses read aloud to the worship songs played.

We wanted our guests to see that we meant our promise. Thanks to God, we were a couple. We were ready to spend the rest of our lives glorifying Him—together.

> *Thanks to God, we were a couple. We were ready to spend the rest of our lives glorifying Him—together.*

The ceremony went perfectly, and the reception did too. A pasta buffet filled up our guests' bellies, as did our strawberry and white wedding cakes. A limo ride for our wedding party made the day feel special, and so did the toasts. We made several hundred dollars during the dollar dance, which we planned to spend on our honeymoon to Disney World. My father-in-law hooked us up with passes. But out of everything that happened that day and night, the dances were some of the most special moments.

There was only one song for Mike and me to dance to, the song that had kicked off the romantic butterflies in the first place, "Godsend" by DC Talk. After we danced, Dad stepped onto the dance floor and took my hand. I nearly started crying.

A host of memories flooded back as we swayed to the song Dad had chosen, "In My Daughter's Eyes." The evening we dropped him off at insurance school two hours away. His insistence on driving straight to the doctor once he found out about my bleeding. Our pillow fights in the Houston hotel room. Our "buggy rides" to all thirty radiation treatments. It felt as if we'd already lived a lifetime of moments together, although I was only twenty-one. In his eyes, I was his baby girl, his Punkin Mary. He didn't need to say it, I knew it was hard for him to give me away.

Mike and his mom danced next, and their song lightened the heavy, emotional mood, but only briefly. Dad took the microphone and announced the next dance, asking for a special friend named Sue. She'd been fighting cancer and had made it her goal to be well enough to dance at my wedding, just like my goal of attending the prom.

"I'd like all the cancer survivors to come down for a cancer survivor dance," Dad requested.

Mike took my hand as we stepped onto the dance floor again. Soon, Mike's grandparents; his aunt and uncle; and Sue and her husband, Mike M., were dancing next to us as "Stand by Me" played. I leaned in to press my cheek against Mike's. I'd never been to a wedding reception with a cancer survivor dance before, but I was thankful to host one at mine. We were the youngest couple on the dance floor by several decades, proudly swaying next to the others. Nick's words were already replaying through my mind. Our story would inspire so many.

Later that evening, cans and streamers clink-trailed behind us as we pulled away. The whole way to the hotel, we talked about our favorite moments. The flowers. The cake. The friends. I couldn't believe it—after five years of dating, we were *finally* married. It was a day I'd dreamed about for so long. An event I'd planned for a year. After the wedding of our dreams, we fulfilled the promises we'd both kept for more than ten years. True Love Waits brought no regrets.

5-7-05

To My Beloved, Danielle,

I have delighted myself in the Lord, and He has brought me to you. God's going to take care of us! You're the best. I am blessed. Thank you for being you! I will love you forever.

—Mikey

As newlyweds, we walked on cloud nine. My ring sparkled. I loved signing my new name, Mrs. Burgess. To help me get comfortable with my new last name, Mike nicknamed me B (which most of our friends started calling me too). I had in-laws! Fun! We made our own holiday plans! At Thanksgiving, I learned how to make green bean casserole. Everything about marriage was awesome. Permanent smiles were pretty much affixed to our faces.

Setting up a home in our two-bedroom duplex was an adventure we'd waited for, though we didn't have a lot of extra money since I was still in college and Mike was teaching. But we didn't care about being poor, and we didn't really see ourselves as such. Our worn-out green futon made a suitable couch. Our fifty-dollar TV was a great deal. All our furniture was either given to us by friends or inherited from our old childhood bedrooms—with the exception of our washer and dryer set, which we bought used off a website for a hundred dollars.

For years, we'd driven back and forth down the highway or hugged in the hallway of my dorm at night. We'd longed for the day when we could roll over in bed and kiss each other good night. Washing our clothes together was an adventure, as was grocery shopping and using our grill. Yes, we'd lived through so much already, yet everyday life had also just begun. Outside of a few newlywed spats, married life came easily.

I graduated college six months after the wedding and started my first job. I'd heard of other young patients going into medicine after they survived a medical crisis, but becoming a doctor or nurse wasn't a good fit. I'd only needed to faint once during a blood draw to learn that working in a field full of needles wasn't a good long-term goal. Upon learning that communications professionals got to write, tell stories, and represent others, it sounded like the best option. After a Kansas City advertising agency offered me a job following college graduation, our dual-income life had blissfully begun.

One year into marriage, we bought a house—very suddenly. Mike saw it first, a 1920s Craftsman bungalow for sale in the downtown area we loved. Buying a house wasn't on our radar, but Mike happened to see the sign, called about it, and after a showing several hours later, we fell in love. The house had everything we wanted; it felt a little too good to be true. It was charming and cozy. There was something special about it. We made an offer right away, since historic houses didn't stay for sale very long in the neighborhood.

We'd not been shopping the market, nor had we toured any other houses, but we had a feeling, the peace of the still, small voice. It was where God wanted us to live. Weeks later, we took hold of the keys. Soon it had a nickname: the Corner of Monroe.

It was more space than we needed for the two of us, but we had big dreams and wanted to welcome others in. We got started right away by adopting two dogs and hosting Sunday night small group. When we joined the team launching a new church (or church planting, as we called it), we opened our house even more. Loud drums and guitars signaled Wednesday night worship practice in the basement. Cars lining the street meant girls' nights, game nights, and prayer meetings. Oven timers were the signal for dinners around the table. The corner seat on our couch became a destination for both new and old friends. The Corner of Monroe was the place to be for New Year's Eve (at least until we began juggling life with kids).

My teenage years had made the American dream (the goal to which we suburbanites seem to aspire) feel far off and unrealistic. But marriage, home ownership, and starting a church from the ground up restored its possibility. If Mike and I were tackling life together, nothing could get in our way.

We assumed we'd lived through the worst of the worst before we ever said "I do." Life would be uphill from here, but we were prepared for any challenge. Fights over toothpaste. Money discussions. Finding patience for an overgrown, weed-filled yard. Balancing multiple families. Hanging the toilet paper roll. Yet we weren't at all ready for the curveball we got, one completely outside our view. We'd promised to love "in sickness and in health," not realizing our "in sickness" days weren't over.

One Heart

Glorify the Lord with me
Let's exalt His name together
We'll sing praises forever
He holds these two becoming one

Hallelujah, Glory
One heart in thee

With our eyes we will look and radiate
Our faces never shamed
Oh, taste the Lord is good
We'll seek Him and lack no good thing

Hallelujah, Glory
One heart in thee

Exalt Your name
As one we'll praise
Exalt the king
As one we'll sing

Hallelujah, Glory
One heart in thee

—Michael Burgess, 2005 (written by Mike for Danielle and performed at the wedding)

PART 3

18

Round 2

"THE GOOD NEWS IS, IT'S stage 1."
My doctor's mouth was moving, but I didn't hear her words. Like a scene out of one of the many sitcoms Mike loved watching, the commotion surrounding the main character (in this case, me, the patient), suddenly got fuzzy and went into slow motion. I heard nothing once "it's cancer again" had been said. It couldn't be. The *good* news? How did I get here? Cancer Round 2?

A sinking feeling hit my already-sore and bandaged stomach—it felt a lot like it did eight years prior when Dr. Connor first operated. I knew the pain well. I'd been here before. But a few things were very different. For starters, it wasn't Dr. Connor talking.

With his sights on retirement, Dr. Connor had introduced his colleague Dr. O'Brien, a surgeon who would soon be taking over his patients. I really didn't like the idea of my doctors retiring and not treating me anymore.

Talk about another hard loss. But if Dr. Connor was insistent on working less, I couldn't have asked for a better replacement. I liked Dr. O'Brien right away, simply because she was female. A girl in proctology? What a treat, even if it meant I needed surgery again.

Her bedside manner was similar to Dr. Connor's, and she was incredibly warm and kind (not to mention beautiful—her white teeth sparkled when she smiled). Dr. Connor reassured us she was artfully skilled and highly respected for her ability to perform laparoscopic surgeries, which meant minimal cutting. She and Dr. Connor agreed I was a good candidate during my pre-op visit. Dr. Connor reassured me *both* of them would perform the surgery. It was hard to believe and I was struggling to process it. Because of a concerning colonoscopy, I was looking at colon surgery again.

With laparoscopic surgery, the expected hospital stay was only a few days. I already knew no surgery is easy, but I felt confident in its relative simplicity and assumed I'd be back on my feet quickly. None of us anticipated the situation that unfolded shortly after the operation— complications with surgery *and* another cancer diagnosis.

I knew I was at high risk for cancer again since I'd already had it once, but for some reason, Cancer Round 2 came out of nowhere. Sitting under warm white blankets with a soundtrack of beeping machines, IV tubes, and Velcro wraps squeezing my legs, I grew very sad. Little did I know, Mike, Mom, and Dad had already gotten tipped off that I'd be facing cancer again. The doctors had pulled them into a small room to explain what they had found. Poor Mike. Mom and Dad were veterans, but this was his first experience. None of them dared to tell me, however, once I woke up and immediately started asking how it had gone. They let the pathology report come back and deliver the news. I can't say I blame them.

Devastated. Angry. Desperate to find the cause, I mentally retraced my steps as though I'd lost something along the way, looking for how and why a second cancer could have happened.

"I've been doing everything I was told to do!" I explained to Dr. O'Brien. I literally wasn't sure what else to say or whom to trust.

Genetic testing showed us I carried some type of gene variant, but its significance was labeled "unknown." Clueless to what the words and letters on the printout meant, my seventeen-year-old interpretation labeled my cancer as (not so scientifically) a fluke. As the years went on and my scans showed up clear, I hit the coveted five-year and seven-year cancer-free milestones. I even got a permanent blue star tattoo (the symbol for colon cancer) on my belly to celebrate. Minimal screening seemed to be a good approach, and I didn't argue with doctors about it.

Devastated. Angry. Desperate to find the cause, I mentally retraced my steps as though I'd lost something along the way, looking for how and why a second cancer could have happened.

My appointments with Drs. Paradelo and Connor had dropped off once I was declared cancer free, and I was down to seeing Dr. Rosen every six months for blood work, CT scans, and x-rays. I visited Dr. Hunter every year for ob-gyn stuff and Dr. Taormina every three years for a colonoscopy. We all assumed this routine would be aggressive enough to catch any sign of cancer's attempted return. Unfortunately, we assumed wrong. I couldn't understand how I'd gone into the hospital for *preventive* surgery and woke up with cancer—again!

A moment from Christmas Eve six months prior had been the impetus, a moment I would have handled differently had I known we were dealing with cancer. Sitting by the window of the guest bedroom at Mike's grandparent's house, I'd taken Dr. Taormina's phone call. I normally wouldn't have answered the phone during a Christmas gift exchange, but I was expecting to hear back about my colonoscopy report. I knew Dr. Taormina was concerned about a polyp he'd removed during the procedure and sent off for testing. When his number popped up on my flip phone, I both marveled at how far technology had grown in a decade (a doctor could call me directly when I wasn't at home) *and* that he cared enough to call personally. Dr. T (as I called him) cared a lot about me as his patient. I liked to think I got the special treatment. Between offering some of his hockey season tickets to Mike and me, inviting us to ride in a convertible during a St. Patrick's Day parade, and then later hiring me to help market his practice, he'd taken a vested interest in my life. I appreciated that—and him.

"The polyp I removed during your colonoscopy came back benign, but I wouldn't take my chances. It looked concerning. I think your cancer may try to return."

He went on to explain his recommendation: to reduce my cancer risk, I needed to reduce the amount of colon in my body. The operation was called a subtotal colectomy, and it would take out nearly all but a foot or so of my large intestine. Since it was clearly the target, fewer feet of colon meant both less area to get cancer and less area to scope. He knew I wouldn't enjoy the idea of surgery again (who would?), but I was reasonable, and I got it.

He was in the midst of reassuring me it wasn't the same thing as an ostomy and that my body would eventually adjust to life with less colon when Mike walked into the room. A pitiful puppy-dog glance told him without any words: it wasn't the worst, yet it wasn't the best, of news. With Mike's hand resting on my knee, I wished Dr. T Merry Christmas and hung up. Mike's arms wrapped around me immediately following and reminded me that the two of us could get through anything. A few days later, I called Dr. Connor's office and got the ball rolling. I journaled to cope.

December 27, 2008
News came on Christmas Eve. I was relived not to hear the c-word again! The scary news is Doctor T is concerned about my rapid polyp growth and

wants to remove most of my colon. Scary surgery, more time off, different lifestyle again. I'm praying for peace and wisdom. I feel like it's the right thing to do in the long run, but I'm concerned about the financial and long-term implications.

I didn't rush into the surgery, partly because of our calendar, partly because I enjoyed feeling in control, and partly because I was loving life and wasn't ready to put it on hold. Unlike the first time I'd experienced doctors telling me to call a colorectal surgeon, I wasn't facing an imminent threat to my life or being told to lie on tables and get poked. As an official adult now, I was running the show. I got to call the shots. So, I held off surgery for six months, not realizing I was living with cancer—again.

The church we'd helped start was growing, and I'd taken a staff role. I'd always wanted to work in full-time ministry, and after an opportunity with our new church presented itself, I couldn't say no. I quit my job in advertising and became the director of communications for our faith community. Helping establish a church name, logo, website, and communications plan was fun, but the relationships that came out of starting a church were the most rewarding. For starters, I was doing it alongside Nick and Leslie. Nick was our pastor. I couldn't believe that from Camp Shamineau to starting a new church, we were still so close.

It didn't take long for Mike's and my nights and

weekends to be spent with buds from the church and neighbors living down the street. Brian and Kelley, two of our closest friends, took road trips with us and hosted movie nights. They too were a dual-income-no-kids couple—otherwise known as DINKS. With friends like them and so many others, adulting was actually fun.

Cancer wasn't an active part of my life, but I occasionally looked for ways to celebrate being a survivor. One day, I found a 5K race benefiting colon cancer in Saint Louis and when my friends heard about it, they wanted to run it with me. The call about surgery had come at Christmas, but the race was planned for March. Since it was an optional, preventive surgery, I didn't cancel our plans. I was experiencing something I'd longed for as a teenager: social support.

Even friends and family members who weren't very athletic wanted to come and run the race. Many of them didn't know me when I'd faced cancer at age seventeen, yet they'd heard the stories. Despite the morning of the race being completely dreadful—bone-chillingly cold, windy, and rainy—we had a blast. The team suited up in ponchos and adhered temporary blue star tattoos on their hands and faces. When we huddled for the camera, I was overwhelmed by their love. I'd received unconditional support from Mike for so many years, but now I also had it from a group of friends. The 5K race was just the beginning of people going above and beyond.

I eventually scheduled surgery with Drs. Connor and O'Brien for June, and my friends continued to rally. My accountability partners Amy and Ashley kidnapped me a few nights before the operation by unexpectedly showing up to my house and wrapping a blindfold around my eyes. They carefully guided me into the car, buckled me up, and drove to an undisclosed location. About ten minutes later, I discovered where they'd taken me as a major "Surprise" erupted once the blindfold came off.

Several of my closest girlfriends had gathered at a local wine bar to shower me with encouragement and fun. *Ting ting!* They lifted their wine glasses to "cheers" my strength. I was so thankful for each one of them. As I received their big hugs, I found my determination. I could face hard things. I thought of them when my hospital stay ran unexpectedly long and complications arrived at every turn. It wasn't hard, my hospital room was often filled with their friendly faces.

Once I finally made it back home, Casserole Nation, as Ashley's husband Danny called it, was in full force. Homecooked meals showed up at our door each night, a flashback to the days when my library coworkers and our church friends cooked for us. But my friends weren't the only ones bringing light and love into a difficult and dark time.

As he sat in the waiting room alongside my parents and extended family, Mike mentioned that our old house lacked an upstairs bathroom and that I'd been feeling anxious about going up and down the stairs postsurgery. Whatever he'd said inspired my aunt Deann and uncle Kenny to take on a quick remodel. Between the morning I was admitted to three weeks later when I got discharged, an upstairs closet had been transformed into a small bathroom with a toilet and sink. I gasped when I saw it. Teary eyed, I didn't know what to say. It reminded me of the closet-turned-bathroom at Grandma Pat's house; the similarity made me smile. The story of Dad and his friend Mike M. working nonstop on the construction especially meant so much. I wondered if Mike M. had quickly jumped in to help as a way to honor his late wife, Sue. She'd passed away not too long after dancing at my wedding. Mike M. hated cancer too.

My Mike loved to surprise me, always, but learning about the bathroom installation while at the hospital was a good thing. It brought sunshine despite the rain clouds called complications. The quick laparoscopic surgery turned into a major ordeal. After I couldn't stop throwing up, both doctors and nurses grew concerned. To understand why, the team needed to open me up. So much for avoiding an invasive operation and shorter hospital stay.

Mike had committed to teaching summer school, which meant he was gone during the days. Since Mom also worked as a teacher but didn't do summer school, she stepped in to stay overnight with me. Although I was now in my midtwenties, it felt nice to be her baby girl. I didn't decline her soothing strokes against my forehead. They helped ease my disappointment and calm me down. Her presence was a reminder I'd been through this once, and God willing, I would get through it again.

I hoped so. I needed to be ready to be a bridesmaid in just a few weeks.

The summer was becoming a perfect storm. If I had known it wouldn't be so quick—*and* I'd be facing cancer again—*and* I'd end up staying in the hospital for nearly a month, I would have forgone the 5K race and scheduled the operation much sooner. But I didn't know that. I assumed June would be fine despite the family weddings planned for July and August. I was wrong.

Andy had gotten engaged, and so had Mike's sister, Laura. My soon-to-be sister-in-law, Ashley, and Laura both asked me to be bridesmaids in their weddings. It was an instant yes to each one! I was excited to not only stand with them during the ceremony and wear beautiful dresses, but for the showers and bachelorette parties. As I sat in the hospital bed with an NG tube in my nose and a tube for nutrition in my arm (some white, chalky stuff called TPN), I kicked myself for my poor timing.

I felt like a failure at managing my own health care. Mom and Dad made it look so easy. In addition to the regret I felt about bringing cancer into a summer that was supposed to be full of happy vacations and beautiful weddings, a looming question wouldn't stop taunting me: *Could I have prevented this if I had scheduled surgery sooner?* When Dr. T stopped by to visit, I straight-up asked him, but he tried to reassure me and take the pressure off.

> I felt like a failure at managing my own health care. Mom and Dad made it look so easy.

"I was concerned right away when I saw the polyp."

Perhaps he was right. He didn't get a cancerous part of the polyp in the biopsy. Or perhaps not. Maybe the polyp turned cancerous during the six months I waited for surgery. But what was done was done. There was no going back and changing it. Fortunately, eventually, I did get better and made it home. My dogs wagging their tails, a brand-new bathroom, a fridge full of meals and groceries thanks to more generous friends—so much goodness awaited me. And after a few weeks, I did make it back onto my feet—in high heels.

"Whoa, you're so tiny!"

Amber rushed across the parking lot to give me an enveloping hug. We'd not seen each other since I'd gone into the hospital, and our long embrace said it all—wow, I missed you, and whoa, what a month!

Laura 's July wedding was taking place at a church not too far from Amber's house, and I welcomed the drive to the country. It sparked memories of good times. Seeing my smiling friend in her fabulous earrings (which I'd begun wearing too, inspired by her) was even more medicine to my weary, yet excited, soul. I appreciated the chance to take deep breaths of the good ole country air again.

I knew I was skinny, but I'd not realized just how thin I looked until Amber saw me. Like a good girlfriend, she flattered me and commented. My smaller size made sense—I was forbidden to eat solid food for most of the three weeks in the hospital while my digestive system was shut down. Dealing with new scars and more frequent bathroom visits was a struggle, but feeling skinny brought joy. I wasn't sure how to handle it.

On one end, I loved the feeling. My heart swelled when Mike's mom offered to take in the sides of my bridesmaids dresses because they'd quickly become too big. A certain freedom came with feeling skinny, probably because I still believed it's what made me beautiful. While I'd come a long way since my elementary days of tossing my lunch in the trash because I thought I looked fat, a small dress size was key to being the perfect woman, or so I told myself.

But my joy of feeling very thin didn't last long. I eventually began eating again. As the family weddings came, I couldn't resist the wedding cakes and other delicious treats. I eventually began to gain back some weight. Yet my constant awareness of the number on the scale was fading away because I had bigger concerns. Unlike everyone else living with between four to five feet of colon, I was now living with one.

To survive not only cancer, but life with a very short colon, I had to accept and try out new diets. If I didn't want to feel miserable or stay stuck inside the house, I had to cut back and even eliminate some food choices. Spicy, fried, and flavorful foods, along with loads of fresh salads, nuts, seeds, and heavy cream, I learned, needed to be eaten minimally. (Fortunately, candy and cookies digested quite easily.) A new relationship with food formed, and it spilled over into my relationship with my body. I was learning to listen to my body, it told me what it could and couldn't handle. I was learning to nurture it, actually wanting to give it care. And I was learning to like it, to appreciate what it had been through. While saying I loved my body still felt like a stretch, my feelings about it were definitely changing.

It wasn't a secret, my body and I had experienced

a love-hate relationship (okay, more hate than love) over the years. It had been too heavy, too curvy, and way too pale beginning back in fourth grade. Never enough, always needing to improve, my body continually failed. The magazines filling my head with a culturally created standard of beauty didn't help, and neither did facing Cancer Round 1. I hated that my body produced cancer, I was embarrassed with the spotlight on my rear.

Yet after Cancer Round 2, something began to change. The flawless image I had hoped to achieve, and the tiny frame I had obsessed about, suddenly didn't seem important. Maybe it was because I was older, or I wasn't consuming so many beauty magazines. Maybe it's because three weeks in the hospital without solid food gave me a new appreciation for eating. But when I truly began to see what my body had lived through, it earned my respect. The fact that it was still standing was remarkable. This new view changed me.

I was learning to listen to my body, it told me what it could and couldn't handle. I was learning to nurture it, actually wanting to give it care. And I was learning to like it, to appreciate what it had been through. While saying I loved my body still felt like a stretch, my feelings about it were definitely changing.

I would have never expected such reconciliation to come from Cancer Round 2. Although a total shock, it was way less life-threatening than Cancer Round 1, and it didn't require harsh chemotherapy. But in a way, Cancer Round 2 was much more life-changing. I felt victory over a fight I'd fought since puberty. Patching things up between me and my body exposed something I couldn't see. My heart, soul, and mind needed some love, too.

19

Promise

AT AGE SEVENTEEN, I DIDN'T know cancer to be a multifaceted disease. When it hit in the middle of my junior year of high school, cancer became one thing: a roadblock in my life as a teen. I'd not processed how cancer made me *feel* (outside of occasionally writing in journals and sharing updates with Mike). When treatment ended, I'd blazed into my next chapter, ready to start bigger and better things.

My testimony was definitely more interesting. (I got to say I believed in God because He helped me fight cancer and I beat it!) I had become living proof of the verse Romans 8:28, which people often liked to quote to those of us who got sick: God had seemingly worked all things together for my good. Yet as Cancer Round 2 entered my story, the same idea that God could use it to spice up my testimony was nearly nonexistent. I didn't quite see it that way anymore.

"Please . . . tell me I'll never get cancer again."

It had been a secret, near-silent prayer coming from one of my dark hospital rooms at age seventeen. I knew I shouldn't test God, but I was hopeful He understood why and what I was asking. The Bible verses said, "Ask and you shall receive." So I asked for a biggie.

"Help me never get cancer again."

It was a bold ask, yet as it rolled off my lips, I could have sworn I heard the still, small voice give a quick God-reply: "You will never get cancer again."

Peace. Warmth. I felt it all immediately in my chest. It was just like many other times when I'd sense God talking to me. I claimed the promise. It was like getting a coveted gift, and I treasured it in my heart for years to come. As my life played out, so did the promise. I was cancer free and healthy. It felt serendipitous when, years after I'd obtained my degree and got some work experience under my belt, doors opened for me to fulfill another long-lost goal: full-time ministry. I left my job in advertising to raise my own financial support and join our church's staff, calling myself an "American mission-ary."

Year after year when the anniversary of my diagnosis rolled around and I remained cancer free, my faith grew stronger. God was keeping His promise. Yet eight years later, when doctors dropped the c-word on me, it felt as though God had broken it.

"I thought He said . . ."

I whispered my question once I got alone with Mike. I didn't want to speak it too loudly, nor in front of our church friends—Danielle, the strong and faithful survivor, the woman in ministry, suddenly questioning God? It felt heretical. Yet Mike knew why I was struggling, and deep down, he was too. Not only had I carried the promise of a cancer-free life from God, Mike believed I'd been fully healed.

"I had a dream in college, when you got sick the first time, where I saw someone being let down and then raised up again . . . and when the person came back up, people celebrated. I felt like this was God's way of telling me you were going to be okay. He's going to heal you."

Neither one of us expected future health problems when we'd waltzed hand in hand into blissful matrimony. For years my promise had played out until one fateful afternoon when it didn't. A second cancer? It was not only a slap in the face but a dart popping an inflated faith balloon.

Did I hear God wrong?

At first, I wondered. Later, I started to negotiate.

Maybe He meant I wouldn't need treatment *again . . . which makes sense. My cancer was stage 1, and we got it all with surgery . . . I don't need chemo or radiation. Maybe* that's *what God meant?*

I wasn't really sure, nor was I able to think or pray through it. Physically, adjusting to my body following surgery was hard. I couldn't really handle what it was doing to me spiritually. As my body settled into a new normal and the scars began to heal, I went straight back into my old life (just as I had gone right back into my senior year) when I got the surgeon's all clear. Pulling up a chair to our planning table, I eagerly engaged in conversations about the upcoming sermon series at church and the children's Bible curriculum. Yet something was different. A nagging question loomed in my mind when we'd bow our heads and pray.

I gave up everything to work for You . . . see? How could You let me get sick again?

Did my long Christian walk count for nothing? Or the way I'd handled Cancer Round 1? Were my journal entries full of prayers and praises not good enough? Or even heard? I was at a loss.

My body had betrayed me. I didn't trust the blood running through my veins. And now, the one thing I'd clung to in my life—God—also seemed to turn His back on me. Ouch.

> *My body had betrayed me. I didn't trust the blood running through my veins. And now, the one thing I'd clung to in my life—God—also seemed to turn His back on me. Ouch.*

I didn't want to blame God, much less argue with Him over this, but over time, I couldn't hold it back. A dam of doubts broke and led me to shelve my Bible except when I *had* to use it for work. I stopped personal quiet times. When people around me prayed, I closed my eyes, but I rarely prayed too. The girl who'd left Camp Shamineau was gone. What I'd found that week, for the first time since then, seemed very far away. Despite what years of journal entries tried to tell me, I didn't believe God was present. I set out to find a new way of coping all on my own. Shattered, I'd lost my faith.

It was unfortunate timing, really, because staying cancer free became a heavier burden, and I could have used the help of a higher power. But just because God and I weren't exactly on speaking terms, it didn't stop my medical carousel from spinning faster.

I was urged to connect with a genetics team (again). My two bouts of colon cancer, at ages seventeen and twenty-five, were suspicious and concerning. A new doctor, Dr. Geier, entered the picture, and fortunately, he made gene defects easy to understand. And he was funny. We expected the testing to come back confirming what doctors suspected—I had a genetic syndrome. Yet once again, the variant was "of unknown significance." But that didn't stop my docs from pivoting. Not wanting to take any chances, I got put on a very high-risk follow-up schedule. With endometrial and ovarian cancer risks also now looming, I began doing more frequent blood work and urine scans. I just wished getting a now-yearly colonoscopy was as easy as checking my pee.

I wasn't doing anything new. I'd done all these tests before, but the increased frequency of them, and the looming threat of another cancer, did make it hard to stay positive. Friends from church were, fortunately, still over-the-top supportive. And while I didn't have much faith of my own, they helped carry me. And they gave me good ideas.

"You should start a blog!"

Blogs were becoming really popular. They were like online journals (made public) where people wrote all kinds of things. Moms blogged, bakers blogged, fashion divas blogged. My friends suggested that as a cancer survivor, I could write one too. I resisted the idea at first, unsure about my ability to do it, and did the world really need one more blog to read? Yet not long after, as I mulled over the suggestion, I decided to give blogging a shot.

November 9, 2009

Welcome to the latest blog about colons. I've created this blog for two reasons.

1. They say it's good to have a place to let off steam. This will be my "dumping spot" for all things colon related. I will be as candid as possible in my stories. I hope people with normal colons will find more appreciation after chomping down that plate full of refried beans without thinking twice, and my fellow semicolons will find comfort that they're not alone—and even laugh with me about what we go through.

2. I love to write. Anne Lamott says to be a good writer, write every day. So my topic of choice, which affects me every day: my colon, or lack thereof. Get ready for tales of the good and the bad. Maybe living through such a dramatic life event will have some rewards in the end. So with

that, welcome to the blog. Let the games
begin . . .

It felt good to hit Publish. When I let Mike know
I'd started a blog, he hollered, "Yeaaahhh, awesome!"
and gave me a big hug. He'd always been so supportive,
including of my writing aspirations. I wasn't sure who
would read my blog, but as I got into a groove of posting, it didn't really matter. Blogging helped me rediscover
what I'd experienced, from the plays in fourth grade to
journals traded with Mike: writing healed.

After only a few weeks, I'd published several posts.
"My Mexican Emergency" tactfully told people about my
full-on restroom dash after eating a spice-filled dinner on
the Plaza. "My PET Scan Experience" explained what
spending four hours at a test that "lit up" cancer cells in
the body was like. I wrote about selecting Thanksgiving
foods as a "semicolon." I gave colonoscopy survival tips.
Over time, the blog helped create meaning for the hard
(and the fun) things I had faced. If I could help someone
else with colon cancer not feel so alone, or a noncancer
patient learn how to relate to someone like me, it was a
bonus.

I kept the blog light (and tried to be funny), since
colon cancer was already so heavy. But one day, the blog
took a vulnerable turn. I wasn't sure how else to cope
with my unexpected phone call but to write.

December 7, 2009
I thought it was strange when I missed three calls
from my oncologist's office this morning. There

were not any messages, but I figured they would call back again. I was right, as I got the call just after lunch. In the cancer community, a phone call can change everything. Especially when it comes from your oncologist's office. Sometimes it's bad news; other times it's good. Today the call wasn't anything that I expected. Val, one of my chemo nurses from many moons ago, was on the phone. She wanted to make sure that I knew. Kim, one of my favorite nurses and people whom I've grown the closest to, was killed in an auto accident last week. She knew I would want to know.

Nurse Kim, a light who had once shone into my darkest of days, was gone. How could this be? My heart ached immediately—another hard loss. It had been just weeks prior when I last saw her. I updated her on my blog, our church, and how I was generally feeling. She was so proud of me. If there was any bright side to Cancer Round 2, it had been that I got to see Nurse Kim more often since I was going to Dr. Rosen's office more frequently. As I gave her updates, she'd share too. A beaming bride, she'd just gotten remarried.

God, why her? How could this happen . . . How are You good?

The life losses were stacking up. Instead of blaming the road conditions or bad weather, I went straight to the source. As I understood it, God had the power to keep cars on the road. Why would He let such an incredible person, someone who cared for thousands of cancer patients and was a survivor herself, be taken so abruptly from this life? It wasn't fair.

My darkened soul grew darker, and my fairly nonexistent faith wanted to collapse. Yet during Nurse Kim's funeral, the legacy of her life challenged my questioning faith.

"Kim let the Lord pull her from some dark pits and we watched as He did put a new song in her mouth and gave her a hymn of praise. It is our prayer that wherever you find yourself today in your relationship with God, you will see from her life that you too can trust in the Lord."

Her sister Cindy was speaking and urging everyone to hang on to hope despite the unfortunate circumstances.

Hope. It was the word hanging off the basket Kim had given me during chemo, a basket that had traveled to college and back with me and now had a place in my home. Hope. It was what Kim embodied each time I told her about how God was opening doors in my life.

"Kim let Jesus love and comfort her . . ." Cindy shared.

My eyes perked up.

I'd assumed Nurse Kim was a Christian, although we never point-blank had that talk. Yet there was no other explanation for her radiant kindness and love. As those who loved her continued to eulogize Kim, I felt my weary heart begin not only to deeply mourn, but soften. Mike put his arm around me as tears streamed down my face. I knew funerals were hard for him too, but I was so thankful he'd come with me. He knew I was struggling with doubt. He was too, a little, although it didn't seem to run as deep. But I didn't want to doubt anymore. I wanted to be that girl, and us that couple, who faithfully trusted God to get us through all things. Hope. I knew that's what my life was missing. While my body had healed up, I wasn't done. It was time to address my heart.

"I feel like a layered cake, there's so much stacked on top of each other."

I was talking with my hands, motioning as though an invisible, delicious cake sat in front of me. Sitting back on the couch, trying to relax, I realized the seating was as comfortable as I'd hoped a therapist's couch could be.

Barbara sat across from me in a swiveling desk chair and nodded as I spoke. I guessed she was maybe ten years older than I was, and seconds after meeting I liked her. From her shirt to her shoes, we had similar styles. As we got talking, she offered both a peace and calmness, yet also grit.

"This probably doesn't make any sense," I said after realizing my vague cake metaphor likely sounded silly.

"It makes perfect sense to me."

What had brought me into her office? Well, where should I start? The church and working in ministry weren't going as I'd hoped. I'd been diagnosed with colon cancer again. I imagined my parents' divorce (although several years ago) and remarriages had something to do with it. Those were just a few of the layers I knew existed.

"I feel crazy."

"You're not crazy . . . although it sounds like what you've lived through could be crazy-making."

I couldn't see it, the hope I'd called her to find. But she seemed to see it hiding under all my cake layers. We started by labeling each one of them "trauma." After one session, I could already feel my heart changing. So I scheduled another. And another.

Eventually, we built up enough trust, and she began saying hard things. "I think you're angry."

"Oh no, I'm not angry." I shook my head right away. She'd been so intuitive about other ways I felt, but suggesting I felt angry? Nope. Not even close. I'd seen anger. It was often a soundtrack to my teenage years. Quiet. Calm. (Yes, even when I got mad.) Those were better ways to describe me.

She smirked and didn't say much, but a few hours later, I realized why.

It happened often after a session. I'd start driving home, and the wisdom of her words, and once-buried memories, seemed to come to mind. It didn't take long this time. She was right. I did feel angry—about a lot of things. Some were obvious (hello, cake layers!), yet others, not so much. When it really boiled down to it, who was I angry at?

God.

"What do I do?" I asked while admitting in our following session she was right: I was angry. I was ready to take the next step.

"You need to be still."

After reciting one line, "Be still and know I am God," from Psalm 46, she got up and left.

I'd never heard of a therapist leaving the room so I could be alone with my thoughts for a few minutes, yet over time, I experienced its power. I felt lighter.

A few nights later, I decided to try the whole "being

still" thing on my own. With Mike away at worship practice, I had the Corner of Monroe all to myself. With my journal and Bible not too far from me, I recited the same Psalm in my mind. But sitting on my bed felt different than a therapist's couch. I fidgeted to handle the weirdness and discomfort.

Rapid thoughts fired through my mind yet eventually slowed when I didn't give up. Eventually, I did start to feel something again. A twinge of hope. Knowing "He is God" led to me opening my Bible not because I *had* to but because I was searching for something. I was looking for God. Where was He? I needed reminding. Thin pages of the New Testament passed through my fingers, and I happened to stop on the Easter story.

"Crucify him!"

I could fairly hear the crowds shouting at a man miraculously healing their bodies (free of charge, even!) because He said He was God's Son. They couldn't accept Him or His message. So they beat Him up. They hammered nails into His hands—something way worse than getting stuck with IV needles. He was offered no painkillers. They then mounted His naked body onto a cross so He'd die. He couldn't even cover up with one of those horrible backless gowns. It was awful.

"I suffered too . . ."

It's amazing I didn't miss it, the quiet whisper that felt more like a long-lost friend. Within seconds, I began to appreciate the faith Mom and Dad insisted I grow up around. Of all of the gods we could have worshiped, of every faith and religion people claimed, no other God did what Jesus did—live a perfect life yet choose to face physical pain. If Jesus was real, if the stories about Him were not fiction but true, He carried enough power to stop His abusers and heal His own wounds, but He didn't.

"Why?"

It was my first genuine prayer after a long season of avoidance. A single word flowed from my heart. The still, small voice brought the answer: you.

Maybe God did promise I'd never get cancer again, but the promise was for a different place, a kingdom with no sickness or death.

While Jesus wasn't only *my* God (He is available to everyone who wants to believe), He became incredibly personal throughout the moments of inner healing. In that space it would have been plausible He died for nobody else but me. The voice challenged me to believe had that been the case, I was still worth it.

I'd always known He died to take away my sins. But I didn't know He suffered so that inside of His scars, I'd find empathy, love, and the courage to trust Him again. When His suffering didn't end in death, I found hope. Because of His risen life, everything started to make sense.

But God said I wouldn't get sick again.

I'd experienced the Jesus story anew and found a deepened, restored faith. But the lingering questions about what had happened to my promise from God stuck around until He helped me see.

Had I heard God *wrong*—He didn't promise I'd never again get cancer? Maybe. It was even possible I wanted to hear those words so badly I convinced myself I'd heard the voice of God and not my own. Or had God really said it but lied to me? Definitely not. As I grappled with the same questions that led to my crisis of faith, a new thought brought peace.

Maybe God did promise I'd never get cancer again, but the promise was for a different place, a kingdom with no sickness or death. A kingdom where Jesus is now, where He rules and reigns.

The Bible backed this up—there's a place of invisible promise. The price of entry? Nothing more than repentance and belief. This new perspective brought comfort. My doubting, wondering heart felt soothed. As I once again put my faith in what my eyes could not yet see, I wondered, *What else could the God of miracles have for me?*

20

September

I'M SURE DR. HUNTER EXPLAINED the specifics about my ovarian suspension surgery prior to starting radiation when I was seventeen, but somehow neither Mom, Dad, nor I fully realized the implications for my fertility until after it was over.

"We don't have time to think about future lives. We must focus on saving her life, now," Dr. Hunter firmly told Dad when he inquired about harvesting my eggs. Fortunately, the docs succeeded—my life was saved, and I eventually made it to adulthood. When Mike and I talked about having a family while we were dating, we knew it wouldn't be a simple feat. His willingness to hold my hand, look into my eyes, and still chose me was still something I struggled to comprehend. How and why did this guy love me so much? I felt so blessed.

"I want to deliver the mail, drive a Jeep, and adopt a toddler."

As a kid, I had three big goals, with adoption being one of them. I'd been interested in adoption after watching our beloved next-door neighbors Dave and Pam adopt their newborn daughter. Eavesdropping on Mom and Pam as they'd chitchat in our front yards, I was intrigued by the idea that a couple could adopt a baby if they struggled to conceive. My Cabbage Patch dolls from way back in the day, who came with distinct adoption certificates, also made adoption feel, well, *special*. As life would bring fertility concerns my way, I offered one response: "Cool. I wanted to adopt anyway."

Yet a few years into newlywed bliss, the situation didn't feel so cool anymore. "Do you think there's *any* chance?" I couldn't help but ask Dr. Hunter during one of our yearly visits.

I knew she'd said, "It's possible, not probable. Yet miracles happen every day" when I asked about birth control a few months before my wedding. I still got periods despite my ovaries being suspended, so I assumed that meant I could still conceive. And while pregnancy wasn't a huge longing of mine, as I planned to adopt no matter what, I became curious about what a "little Mike and Danielle" would look like, especially as we watched our friends and family go through it.

I'd taken Dr. Hunter at her word and began taking birth control pills; even a miracle situation wasn't in Mike and Danielle's initial plans. Yet after a few years, I didn't only want to avoid the monthly prescription expense, I was more open to an improbable situation actually happening. Heck, if my case of colon cancer was a 1 percent likelihood of cases, then a natural pregnancy? We had a good chance!

I began learning about tracking a cycle, and Mike joined the club of husbands who didn't mind one bit that their wives wanted to "start trying." One month, my period seemed late, and I joined the ranks of other women who snuck into a store to nonchalantly buy a pregnancy test. Yet after peeing all over my hand (I'm a gal—I can't aim!), I frowned at the dreadful stick.

"Negative." The blood that followed a few days later didn't help anything. I'd always hated that sight. What a bummer.

"You could call a reproductive specialist," Dr. Hunter said during the next yearly follow-up when she noticed I'd discontinued my birth control prescription. She reassured me I wasn't out of options, but if I wanted to get pregnant, I likely needed help.

I tucked the number of her referral into my pocket, but grief and flashbacks stopped me from making the call.

I couldn't fathom sitting on crinkly-paper-covered tables and facing more needles, stirrups, and shots. I'd watched Kristi go through some of that and wasn't sure I could do it. Knowing I was infertile and likely never going to see birth firsthand, our friend Kelley invited me to her OB appointments as well as into her delivery room. Watching her birth Ella from across the room and hearing a baby's first cry was an incredible moment I couldn't believe I'd witnessed. The beautiful gesture of our friends inviting me into a precious moment had shown me both the miracle of life and how much time was spent in hospitals.

Although I *could* have pursued and checked to see if my ovaries and radiated pelvis were viable for pregnancy,

I lacked peace that fertility treatments were right for *us*. Mike didn't disagree. We'd known infertility was our reality since the day we said "I do." What I didn't know, however, was that I'd eventually *want* to get pregnant. The circumstance had gone from no big deal to painful, and it was yet another layer on my cake, *another* trauma.

Fortunately, Barbara had taught me that to work through the pains of life, there was no way other than through them. I knew that if I wanted to be genuinely happy with my circumstances and glad for others, I needed to make some space and give myself time to heal. It sounded good and easy, but actually doing it was very hard.

I'd need to turn down baby shower invitations because I couldn't handle both the sadness and jealousy when I'd see other women who could "look at their husbands and get pregnant."

I struggled with anger too. My body effortlessly produced cancer, but not human life. It seemed so unjust. Yet as I rode the waves of grief, mourning a life I'd never give, over time, I reached the wave of acceptance. Eventually, Mike and I were ready to revisit our family-building plans.

We knew domestic adoption would be our route to parenthood because Cancer Round 2 markedly changed our plans. We had been exploring international adoption from Ethiopia before I went in for surgery. In addition to feeling a call to adopt, I also kept imagining us with becoming a mom, I didn't picture myself with a white child. I figured it was a clue to guide our path. The quiet whisper agreed.

Cancer Round 2, well, it took international adoption out of the running. Most agencies wouldn't work with us until I was five years cancer free (again). Although we caught my latest cancer early, at stage 1, I technically didn't meet their requirements. Frustrated? For sure. But I trusted there was another plan. I began journaling and praying for our future baby.

About a year after my diagnosis, we'd rebounded and were back to normal life again, or whatever you call life without cancer and unexpected hospital stays. Mike and I agreed to pursue domestic adoption and happened to find an agency that required I be only one year cancer free. It was perfect! Now we just needed to send in our application. I was ready! But . . . Mike was not, or so it seemed. He disliked his teaching job and seemed burdened with decisions about what would come next. When he'd come home at night and we'd find ourselves with nowhere to go, I'd want to talk about adoption planning, but he wanted to grab the remote and flip through TV channels. It was hard. I didn't want to nag, but I was really ready to start talking about adoption. For some couples, I knew their adoptions came after *years* of waiting. I wasn't asking for a baby tomorrow, but I did hope we could have some type of plan to become parents within the decade.

"Mike will know."

A gentle nudge I'd felt during a quiet time cooled my jets and got me to slow down. While I'd always been an ambitious go-getter who liked to make things happen, I did love it when Mike took the lead. And when it came to starting our adoption, I needed to be okay with waiting on Mike. I stopped bringing it up and found contentment. I offered to babysit for our friends to get my baby fix. I also kept writing in a journal to Future Baby B, as I found writing to be therapeutic and help me share (hopeful) mother's heart feelings.

God is bringing you to us at just the right time, He has stirred my heart already!

We're praying about when to start this process. We don't want to be too early or too late!

I know it's up to Jesus. You'll be here when it's your time. Because you will be here for a purpose, you will be sent by God. You're not ours to begin with; He's got awesome plans for you. I've already been praying. So I will sit tight and wait.

The day had arrived! We'd gotten the call. On a fall September afternoon, Mike's sister, Laura, and her husband, Jake, let us, Aunt B and Uncle Mikey, know our niece was born! A few days later, we excitedly drove to southern Missouri to meet her. I looked forward to getting that baby into my arms. A newborn in the family intensified my ache and hopes to become a mom. I too wanted a baby of our own to cuddle and hold.

I'd promised to not bring up adoption with Mike, yet a three-hour car ride was challenging it. An hour and a half in, I miserably failed.

"So . . . any thoughts on starting our adoption?"

Quiet. More quiet. I grew anxious for Mike's response. Missouri farm fields and gas stations zoomed by. To cope with the awkward pause, I looked for the Amish horse-drawn buggies on the side of the road.

"September."

Ah, he spoke. Wait . . . what? "Like . . . *this* month?"

"Yeah."

He'd always been a man of few words. Ever since the day I met him in my driveway, he didn't say a lot. But even I was surprised, after ten years into our relationship and five years married, that he offered such a short response. Not only was it one word, but September was already halfway over! I didn't need to ask for more details. He could tell from my crossed arms and perturbed face that I was annoyed, and he needed to keep talking.

"When I was leading worship at camp this past summer, I took a walk in the woods and was praying about when to start. I felt like I heard the word 'September.'"

I felt all sorts of things, amazingly, in that one second. First, how could he not tell me? That had been more than a month ago! Yet I was too excited to be frustrated very long. September—it was like the magic word I'd been longing to hear. September it was! I nearly floated, in a good way, through the visitor door of the maternity ward.

"Do you have something to tell me?"

I looked down at the text message from our friend René, who was staying at our house to watch our dogs while we were gone. I hoped everything at the house was okay.

"No, why?"

"Are you pregnant?"

I laughed when I saw her message, although it wasn't exactly funny. She knew I was sensitive about infertility, though, and she wouldn't be asking for no reason. I told her the truth.

"No, I'm not pregnant." (I left out the part where Mike and I had just decided to start the adoption process.)

"Oh, okay. I had a dream . . ."

And then our conversation ended.

A few months later, I posted a blog announcing, "We're adopting!" and René texted again. She'd written us a letter after she'd had her dream and told me to save it.

"Open the letter."

I raced downstairs to find it and tore in.

Come to find out, the weekend she stayed at our house, she dreamed of me sitting in a rocking chair in the guest room, which had become a baby's room, with a baby girl in my arms. A couple of dogs were near my feet, and one of them was black.

Her timing had been uncanny, and I was excitedly hopeful for how everything would play out. I tucked the note away and turned to my new focus: adoption paperwork.

Excited and ready to become parents, we most definitely were. But not in a hurry. Unlike some couples facing infertility, ours wasn't unexpected or surprising. I was thankful to get the process started, but I didn't mind the wait. Based on our agency's estimated timetables, the soonest we'd be parents was May—which sounded great. By the end of September, we'd officially submitted our paperwork and planned to take our time throughout the fall. We had many worksheets to complete and visits to schedule with a social worker for our home study. And we were looking for grants.

Funding was a major piece to the adoption puzzle, and honestly, it almost stopped us from proceeding. Mike's meager teaching job and both my job at the church and budding freelance business were paying our bills, but we weren't exactly rolling in the Benjamins—at least not enough to flat-out cover upward of $20,000–$30,000 in adoption costs. Yet our friends Scott and Patti had also adopted, and they began mentoring us every step of the way. The first time we ate dinner together, they reassured us, "If God has called you to adopt, He will provide financially." I sure hoped so.

We looked into special adoption loans and financing, as well as dozens of adoption fundraising ideas. Yet we also mentioned the possibility of asking to borrow money from our parents, and as soon as they all heard about it, they overwhelmingly said yes. Mike's folks, my dad and stepmom, and my mom and stepdad all wanted to help make our dreams of parenthood come true. It was humbling, yet we felt so loved. They didn't only generously offer to help us, but down the line, none of them let us pay them back.

Thanks to our parents' generosity, our savings, and surprise gifts from friends and family, we quickly had a big chunk of the funds we'd need to adopt lined up. I figured God would make a way for the rest to eventually trickle in. And boy, did He.

I'd applied for a grant through a nonprofit organization called the Samfund, which I'd stumbled across one day when searching for adoption funding. The organization existed to help young adult cancer survivors cover the cost of either cancer or rebuilding their lives, adoption expenses included. I gathered up Mike's and my tax information and wrote snippets of our story. We submitted our application for a "family-building grant," and not long after, I was floored to receive a call from the founder, Sam, personally.

"Danielle? This is Sam with the Samfund, and I'm excited to say our board has chosen you as one of our grant recipients!"

I nearly dropped the phone. Get out.

"We're covering the cost of your home study."

I sat in the chair, speechless. "Wow, I'm honored . . ." I didn't know what to say. Getting emotional had never been a strong suit of mine, and I rarely cried. Yet as I hung up with Sam, I couldn't deny I felt a few tears. Maybe the emotions of a hopeful mother were already kicking in; I did notice moms cried a lot. But even more than that, as I took time to take it in, I realized that cancer was finally giving back.

For all my life, cancer had taken things away. My colon. My junior year of high school. Most of my hair. And my fertility. Yet this time, thanks to cancer, I was actually receiving. When Mike got home from school, I shared the news, and we celebrated with takeout pizza and ice cream.

We appreciated that the grant would cover our home study costs, for sure, but it was even more valuable because of what it meant. Cancer had been such a negative to our lives, but it was starting to bring beautiful things. No longer was the disease a big, bad guy lurking in the wings trying to steal my life. The grant kick-started a new way of seeing cancer—more like a trailhead leading us up a challenging path, not so we could jump off a cliff, but take in some majestic views.

"Brrrrr."

I kept repeating myself from the time I closed the car door to the moment the automatic doors to the birthing center opened and we stepped into another hospital lobby. There were only a few reasons I would have left the comfort of my cozy, warm home on a freezing January night (to go to a birthing center, of all places!): meeting a new baby girl from small group. As our group's leaders, Mike and I took our roles seriously. We were shepherding a flock, as church called it. Or to us, we were simply trying to be good friends.

We stomped our feet to shake off the salt from the parking lot. Locating the right room, we knocked once and saw our friend's head peek out.

"She's eating."

Both Mike and I froze, did a 180 turn, and headed for the visitor's area. Say no more. As we settled into maroon chairs across from each other, I looked around the room and read flyers about car seat safety and lactation support groups.

"Just think—we'll be sitting in a waiting room like this in a few months, but the baby back there will be ours!"

Mike didn't offer much of a reply other than a "I know. Weird, right?" look. I instantly felt squeamish. Something about that idea didn't sit well.

"She's done eating. Come on down!"

We didn't plan to stay long, but we—I mean *I*—did want to hold the baby and congratulate our friends. As we were commenting on her tiny hands and getting the lowdown on the first forty-eight hours as new parents, my phone started vibrating across the room. Once we made it to the parking lot, I checked my messages.

"Meet before church in the a.m.?"

It was Scott and Patti.

Now several years into starting our church, we assumed the reason for their text. It was normal by now for friends to drop off and find other places to worship. Yet as we sat across from them in the hotel lobby the next morning (our church rented the ballroom for services), what came next was a major surprise.

"We know this may not be what you're expecting . . . but here's the story. Our friend Nick is taking care of his three-month-old niece right now, and he may be open to adoption. If he is, are you interested, would you want us to share about you with him?"

Oh . . . this was *not* what I was expecting.

I looked over at Mike, and when we made eye contact, I could tell he felt the same thing. Because our infertility had been widely known, we'd already been pegged as prospective parents for a few crisis pregnancies. They'd all fallen through, and we'd learned to not place any hope or expectation in private adoptions. That was one reason we'd gone with our big adoption agency—we felt a little more protected. But we trusted Scott and Patti, and as fellow adoptive parents, they weren't messing with us. We knew they took adoption opportunities very seriously.

Yet I still felt uneasy and unsure, not only because it was private but because the baby lived in town—about ten minutes from us. We'd not fully known how open adoption worked, but if this worked out, it would be more open than both of us initially presumed. Yet I couldn't shake the awkward feeling from the maternity waiting room from the night before. Something about the scenario didn't feel right.

"Sure, we're open."

What else could I say? Both Mike and I were trying to ride adoption's waves. The timing did seem to fit with our process, well, sort of. Our home study had just completed, and we were one round of edits away from finalizing our profile sheet—the one expectant mothers would view to see our photo and learn about our home, community, and parenting philosophy. Once that step finished, we'd go active with our agency and see where it took us.

The clock signaled it was time for services to begin in the ballroom. Before leaving the lobby, Scott said, "Want to see a picture?"

Mike shook his head no, but I leaned in. An adorable little girl was tightly swaddled in blankets and sleeping in a green Pack 'n Play. She looked like an angel baby, from what I could tell. I quickly smiled, let out an "Ahhhh," and then looked away. I couldn't get attached.

"Oh, and she's biracial."

Scott had nearly forgotten that one detail. I wrinkled

my forehead and paused. Really? Biracial? Maybe there was something to this after all.

"I have unbelievable news!" Scott called in a hurry the next morning. He was always calm and easygoing. His excitement tipped me off to something really big.

"Nick called early this morning. I've been praying for him, and we've had lots of faith talks. Last night Nick had an incredible God moment in the middle of the night as he was feeding the baby. He called me this morning and said he wants to talk about adoption."

I couldn't make this stuff up even if I tried.

A few phone calls later throughout the rest of the morning, it seemed the train had left the station.

"Scott called to say Nick wants to meet and talk about us adopting this baby . . ."

I had never called to pull Mike out of his classroom in five years of teaching, but this was a special circumstance. I couldn't handle this news alone, and just like every other major milestone since age seventeen, Mike needed to be a part of it. How could it be happening—already? We both didn't know. Adoptions usually took months, if not years, of waiting. We hadn't even gone active, much less waited one day. Yet although the timing seemed off, we were oddly, somewhat prepared.

Brimming with excitement, each of our parents had not only helped fund the adoption but given us gifts for baby. A white crib and matching changing table and dresser had transformed our guest room into a nursery. At

Christmas, we'd opened gifts tagged Baby B and started loading up on bottles, toys, and a few stuffed animals. I'd assumed the soonest we'd use them was spring, certainly not within weeks. Yet with our lightning-speed pace unfolding, I started to reorient my thinking.

Adoptions usually took months, if not years, of waiting. We hadn't even gone active, much less waited one day.

The next week was full of lots of phone calls and a meeting with Nick. It did feel like a relief when the process slowed down, even for a few days, when we realized Nick wasn't the decision maker. It was his sister, the baby's mom. Nick was confident she'd heed his advice and be on board. While waiting to find out, I called our adoption agency with a heads up—we might have a change of plans.

To our relief, it was no problem. They could facilitate the adoption for us should we get privately matched. The kicker? Should we be reclassified to a private adoption, we already had 100 percent of the funds, the costs were more than cut in half. Wow.

This could really be happening. And that was confirmed when Scott called to say Nick's sister agreed. Adoption was best for her baby. It would give her daughter the life she wanted her to live. I hung up the phone. *Wait—we have a daughter now too? Really?* It was exciting, yet confusing. A few hours later, though, we got yet another phone call with a . . . well, let's call it speed bump.

Somewhere in the mix of Nick and his sister agreeing to pursue adoption, *she'd* called an adoption agency, who quickly met privately with her and arranged for her to meet some of their prospective couples.

"We've got a situation. Can you meet at Nick's tomorrow night?"

Scott filled me in on everything and insisted Mike and I show up at Nick's house after the other agency and prospective couple left. I didn't like the idea of it becoming some type of popularity contest (those days belonged in high school), but we were willing to do just about anything.

The unease made my stomach do roller-coaster moves and flips. We expected the twists and turns—all adoption stories came with them—but this seemed a little extreme. Maybe because it was happening *so fast*. A little more than one week prior, we'd met Scott and Patti in the hotel lobby and agreed to explore the idea. Now we were on a fast track to adopting the baby we'd discussed, and I found my mind trying to think of her as our daughter. I usually processed slowly and needed a lot of time to make decisions. Yet parenthood (or the prospect of it) was already changing me. A week was all I needed to go from guarded and cautious to all in.

"Ready? Let's go." Mike and I agreed to show up as Scott suggested. I prayed that however things turned out, each of us couples would be called Mommy and Daddy one day.

Armpits soaked. Adrenaline pumping through my body. Carefully trying to not slip on the ice that wouldn't seem to melt, I took Mike's arm escorting me to Nick's front steps. I couldn't really tell how Mike felt. Giddy, cautious, yet also excited? We were a mess. I mean, very put together (or so we needed to appear).

Nick must have heard crunching ice beneath our shoes because before we knocked, he was opening the front door. "Come on in. There she is."

Stepping into Nick's entryway, we rubbed our hands to warm up and removed our coats. Scott and Patti waved from the kitchen table, which overlooked the living room in Nick's open floor plan. Although it was Scott's birthday, they'd rushed through their angel food cake tradition so we didn't have to experience the incredibly awkward, yet important, moment with strangers alone.

Taking a seat on the couch, I saw her in the corner of my left eye, but I tried not to stare. A precious baby girl was sleeping in her pink pastel bouncer, cozied up inside a newborn-sized sleeper.

Is that my daughter?

I wanted to look at her, to walk over and cup her little fingers in my hand or gaze at each one of her tiny ten toes. But then I remembered: this wasn't *my* baby. She belonged to the woman in the recliner—a woman whose emotions I couldn't even begin to fathom. Out of respect to the birth mom, I smiled at the baby yet walked past her to take a seat on the couch. Keenly aware that no decisions had been made, I wanted to get to know this brave woman.

"What do you like to read?"

How to start a mammoth conversation like the one we were about to have? Well, I decided to start with books, and fortunately, she did like to read. After talking about the books we enjoyed, I learned she also liked drinking tea. And cats—really, all animals. I felt relieved when our conversation made her rock back and smile. Okay, good. She's relaxed. While the situation at hand could have put us on opposing sides of an invisible line, we weren't all that different. She was just a couple of years younger than me (definitely not the stereotypical teenage birth mom), and she had a good handle on her desires for her daughter.

Although the pregnancy was unplanned, there was no other option in her mind than for her to deliver. The story of what led to us discussing adoption, I promised to keep private and confidential. But as her love and concern for her daughter became evident, so did her courage to share her with us. Few people carried that kind of strength. She earned my instant respect.

Cries from a hungry baby turned our attention to the one reason we'd gathered in Nick's living room.

"Do you want to feed her?"

Nick was shaking a bottle; he'd anticipated she'd wake up hungry soon. I wanted to say yes, of course! I also wanted to say no; it's not time for that yet. But before I could answer, the baby was resting in my arms, and her big brown eyes were already reaching into some of the deepest places of my longing mother's heart. I nearly exploded, yet I tried to stay cool. It was such an odd moment to be experiencing while sitting on a stranger's couch.

I had experience. I'd fed dozens of church friends' babies their bottles, and I hoped I looked like a natural (and impressed them) as the hungry girl gobbled her milk and let out a hearty burp. Mike had stayed pretty quiet during the whole thing, relying on me to carry the conversation yet chime in with eye contact and "Uh-huh" verbal affirmations.

"Do you want to hold her?" I asked Mike, but he shook his head no and declined. Between the two of us, he was actually the more emotional one. Initially frustrated that he wasn't all in like me, I had to remember one fact he didn't forget: she wasn't ours yet.

After we'd been there an hour, Mike's and my non-verbal cues agreed it was time to leave, but before we stood up, Nick offered to take a picture. Mike had already captured one of me feeding the baby, but another one? Of the three of us? *Gahhhh*. More hard things and conflicting emotions! But I took a cue from my own mom, who'd made sure to capture major and minor moments of Andy and me growing up.

Should the three of us become a family, I'll want this picture one day, I told myself. *If not, I'll delete it.*

Heavy. It had been a heavy evening. I felt hopelessly unprepared yet also aware that in life, parenting, and especially adoption, there was no how-to manual. We thanked Nick and his sister for inviting us over, gave a special nod to Scott and Patti, who'd been watching the whole thing, and just as I was about to put on my coat, a black dog walking up the stairs caught my eye.

"This is Miss Bear," Nick said as he scratched behind the ears of his fluffy, bear-cub-sized dog. In an instant, I remembered. René's dream! The room turned into a nursery! The baby girl swaddled in pink! The black dog! It was all making (sort of) sense.

"Can I get a photo with the baby and the dog?" I

asked, willing to risk looking crazy. I didn't have time to explain it, but I knew I would later. I couldn't wait to live out the rest of the story.

By early the next morning, I woke up to an unread email from a new sender. It was the birth mom.

"Mike! Come here!"

With a toothbrush in his mouth and his white undershirt tucked into his jeans, he quickly came, assuming something was wrong. "What? What's wrong?"

"I've got an email from her already."

We both opened our eyes really wide and stared at each other for a second. I assumed our hearts were beating in unison—very quickly.

"I think you'll make great parents for my daughter."

Mouth agape, toothpaste trying to inch down his face, Mike clearly was shocked. His outward expression matched my inward feelings. Wow. Holy cow. We were parents! Wait—we were parents? It was so exciting. And bizarre. Wow, God, just wow.

We reread the email together and then sat on the edge of our bed embracing each other, trying to let it sink in. A few minutes later, I walked downstairs to find Amber. She'd driven up for the weekend to attend my shower. Amy and Ashley insisted it wasn't technically a baby shower since the adoption agency discouraged us from such parties until we were at home with a baby. But an "activation celebration" seemed to be okay, especially the party my friends dreamed up. The girls-only evening would be full of Thai food and wine, gift cards for when we "got the call," and a homemade mobile to hang over Baby B's crib. They knew me well—some of my favorite things, and it was actually a little healing to get thrown a nontraditional baby shower serving alcohol.

Amber knew about our evening prior. I couldn't keep it from her when we came home. When I told her about the email—it was official!—she squealed, gasped, and covered her mouth. All of us in the house were simply dumbfounded. I still needed to talk to our agency and make sure social workers and lawyers were getting lined up. I held off breaking the news to anyone else, but later that night with the girls, I smiled extra wide as we said cheers to Baby B. I had tipped some of them off to a potential new plan forming. Mike was out on the town with a friend watching football and trying to comprehend it. Our moms knew, as did just a few of our friends. The details about Baby B were forthcoming and made public sooner than anyone at the party imagined.

We quickly got ready thanks to Target runs, shopping for a nursery chair with Mimi (what Amy wanted to be called!), and preparing our house for a baby. Dozens of friends replied to our email updates with messages of congrats, gifts, and parenting advice. Mike's mom sewed the nursery bedding. We picked out a colorful pattern with trees. My mom stocked us up with books and outfits. My stepmom quickly offered to help watch her since she ran an in-home daycare. On the evening of January 23, ten years after my parents came to the library to say "You have cancer," I was with them again, yet under wildly different circumstances. Nick generously opened his house for all of Mike's and my parents to meet the baby. They beamed at the sight of their new granddaughter and took turns taking pictures. One by one, amazingly, pieces fell into place.

Three weeks after we sat around a small table in the hotel lobby with Scott and Patti, we sat at another table, except this time in front of a judge. We swore to love the little girl sleeping in her car seat as our own. They didn't call them vows, but the agreements sounded the same. We were ready to become a family, no turning back. Grateful for the government's formalities and caution to place the baby in a safe, healthy home, the judge made official what we already knew in our hearts. God had put together our family. She was ours to raise.

From the beginning of our new family, we had no plans of discontinuing our new relationship with her birth family. Although the time from that first call had only been three weeks, we had totally enjoyed meeting Nick; his daughter, Isa; his sister; and his parents. They'd all played a role in caring for our daughter until she made her way to us. Our families were excited for us without a doubt, but it surprised me when soon the birth family actually became our biggest cheerleaders.

Grateful—we were all so grateful for one another. And we were all committed to doing what was best for our girl. Yet the first thing Mike and I knew we must do once the judge ruled that she now was our child was change her name.

Her birth mom had given her a beautiful name. I loved it. But as her parents, we wanted to follow in the footsteps of biblical figures who got new names as their lives changed. We named her Mae.

To us, Mae stood for new beginnings. (We'd gotten married in the month of May.) It alluded to spring growth—the green and pink that popped up after winter left everything barren. Mae also happened to be the name of Mike's and my favorite band, whose songs eerily paralleled our lives. One day early on in our relationship, we were singing along, and it was like the idea hit us both at the same time. If we got to raise a little girl, she would be our Mae.

What. A. Whirlwind. I could hardly fathom it. For the first time maybe ever, I felt thankful for an ice storm. Just as we made it home from the courthouse, thick ice blanketed Kansas City. After a brief dinner where all our parents, and Mike's grandma, came to snuggle the baby, we got iced in for the next several days. It was serendipitous timing.

Mike, now fully enveloped in full-on dad mode, scooped up our little four-month-old bundle of joy and immediately started bouncing, singing, and chilling on the couch with her. We'd take turns holding and feeding her, as well as learning how to change her diapers and get her to sleep. We'd occasionally look back and forth across the room as the baby slept in one of our arms and shake our heads in wonder.

Every paper had been signed. Every appointment made. Every decision was decided at just the right time. I couldn't help but stand amazed. Out of everything

If we got to raise a little girl, she would be our Mae.

I couldn't help but stand amazed. Out of everything bad that had happened in my life, this little girl was beauty from the ashes. My greatest gift, I called her. I had goose bumps each time I'd think about what had fallen into place so our adoption dreams could come true. Still, nothing gave me more goose bumps than this: we adopted her in January, but Mae had been born in September.

21

Advocate

"Tips to prevent cancer again in young colon cancer survivors."

It probably looked like I was breaking my own advice.

"Don't rely on the internet for your medical answers . . . call a doctor."

Out of the many media interviews I'd done to share my story as word got out about my unlikely path into adulthood, I urged people to not make the same mistakes I had. If they saw symptoms, don't let "Dr. Google" diagnose you. Call a doctor.

But I wasn't typing in my symptoms when I hopped online. I was looking for how to *prevent* symptoms from even occurring. I was desperate to do anything to prevent cancer's return. I wondered if there was any research that could help me know what to do, and I knew that finding my answer would require logging online.

I'd come a long way since my first brush with the internet. As much as I disliked it, in a way, we'd grown up together. Computers appeared in homes around the same time my body went through the changes of puberty. In the decade that followed my development into womanhood, computers—and then wireless technology—also blossomed. Most people I knew were connected through mobile phones and social media by the time I'd reached thirty. As I watched technology boom, I wondered if facing cancer at age seventeen would have been easier, or at the very least, less lonely. If more of my classmates could have seen my Instagram photos from chemo or been able to tweet me a get-well message or post on my Facebook wall, maybe I would have been able to tell a different story. Maybe I would have known to speak up about blood in the stool sooner.

Either way, I'd found a way to embrace going online despite it getting off to a rocky start with the naughty website in elementary school. All sorts of credible groups, from doctor's offices to hospitals and the National Cancer Institute, were putting information about diseases and health on the internet. One night between Cancer Round 1 and Cancer Round 2, fears about recurrence hit, and I logged online.

There are a lot of studies about how to cure cancer. I wonder if I can do anything to prevent it. I typed a variation of my question into the search bar, and a results page full of links quickly generated. One website in particular caught my attention.

"The Colon Club—young colon cancer survivors."

I clicked to view the page, and once it loaded, I saw

a bold picture of a female who looked around my age holding up her shirt to expose a long, vertical scar.

What? Who is this? Did she have colon cancer too?

I quickly searched the homepage for answers and found out I was looking at a project called the Colondar, a calendar of young colorectal cancer survivors. Whoa. I clicked around and found thumbnails of dozens of other men and women lifting their shirt tails to expose a matching scar—and their stories.

I thought I was one of the only ones.

With the exception of an email pen pal named Wendy that M. D. Anderson Cancer Center connected me to, I didn't think any other young colon cancer survivors existed. I'd been told I was one of the youngest survivors in the country. I'd hardly met any other colon cancer survivors in general, and certainly none were my age at the time—or even under fifty. What was this Colondar? I had to find out!

My quest for prevention was replaced with a hunger to read all of these people's stories. I soon gathered I was hardly the only one, and not even the youngest person, to get diagnosed with what many considered "an old man's disease." These people were in their twenties, thirties, and forties. There were even a couple of survivors diagnosed in their teens like me!

In the right-hand corner of the website was a button to join the Colon Club—apply to be in the calendar. I wanted to, but I wasn't ready. I clicked around some more.

Erika, as I'd come to learn her name, was the gal whose abdomen I first saw. A stage 4 survivor from Pennsylvania who'd been diagnosed in her early twenties, she'd come up with the idea of the calendar to raise awareness so people would know colon cancer happened at younger ages too.

She'd pitched her idea to the cofounders of the Colon Club, Molly and Hannah, at a traveling exhibit in a shopping mall that came with mega-props called the Colossal Colon. The crawl-through replica of the human colon was a crazy idea hatched by Molly, another survivor diagnosed at age twenty-three, who as an athlete carried the Olympic Torch. She in turn was challenged by *the* Katie Couric (the *Today* TV anchor who—after losing her husband to colon cancer—went on to broadcast her own colonoscopy in real time) to find a way to raise more awareness. Voila—the Colossal Colon!

Molly was doing all this in honor of her friend Amanda, Hannah's cousin, who'd died of colon cancer, leaving behind two young kids. People, young people, were dying from a preventable disease, but many doctors weren't taking them seriously. I'd never been more grateful for Dr. Taormina in my life. He'd not hesitated to do a colonoscopy when I was seventeen. He was one big reason I was still alive.

Memories of reading over printouts with Mom assuming my symptoms could only mean hemorrhoids flashed back. Nowhere had any information we found said blood in the stool happening in a younger person *could* indicate something serious—especially not cancer. Yet that was *my* story and the stories of dozens of others on this website. Before I logged off the computer, I'd decided to apply.

I looked down at my vibrating phone to see an incoming call from an unknown New York number flashing. I had no clue who it might be.

"Hello, is Danielle there? This is Molly McMaster from the Colon Club. We wanted to invite you to be in our next Colondar! We think you'd be a great! We will take care of everything to get you here—the flight, food, where you stay. If you don't want to travel early in the morning because it's hard on your gut, tell us. We'll get you a late flight. We can't wait to meet you!"

Wait, what? Oh yeaaah, the calendar. Wait, this is Molly? *The* Molly? *I'd* been chosen for a calendar? To be a *model?* Ho-lee-cow. I took rapid notes.

Telling Mike about the call later that night was wicked fun. With fists in the air, he hollered, "Yeah!" I think he was pumped to have his wife be a model. Needless to say, he wanted me to do it. So I said yes. A few months later, I boarded a plane to Albany, New York, and then rode in a limo with a few other survivors into a small lakeside community in upstate New York, a town called Huletts Landing, on Lake George.

"Welcome to the Adirondacks!"

I'd never heard of this part of the country, but I was fairly familiar with their namesake chairs. There were plenty of them sitting on the white porch wrapping the Victorian-style house: our shared destination. It was as if I'd stepped into a real-life postcard, so picturesque—a glass-blue lake full of rippling waves was surrounded by mountains covered in Christmas trees. I still couldn't believe I'd just come on an all-expenses-paid trip to travel here.

I'd been chosen to model for the fifth calendar, and this home, Molly's parents' house, was Colondar headquarters. It was where all the meals were prepped and the photo shoots staged. As for our lodging, we were staying in the guest homes of the neighbors—friends of Molly's family who'd offered their hospitality as a way to support both her nonprofit and personal fight.

From the second I stepped out of the limo, I was mistaken for a celebrity. Colon Club staff and volunteers all knew exactly who I was, and they were so excited to meet me. Not even at church had I been welcomed so fondly. It was overwhelming yet, after I warmed up to it, fun.

"How was your trip? Where do you live again? Look at your long, gorgeous hair! Tell us your story—you were seventeen, right?" They'd really done their homework, which helped break the ice. They'd also studied the other eleven models who were going through a similar experience. I'd soon spend many days and nights getting to know them, learning how our stories were both similar and worlds apart. It was interesting, but not in a bad way. As one of the youngest at the shoot, and the youngest to be diagnosed, I was still one of the furthest out from diagnosis. My short life and story was giving older, wiser survivors hope.

Although the shy side of me came out, it was a lot to take in, I enjoyed meeting everyone over the week, especially my roommate Libby. We were the "two young ones," as everyone called us, still in our midtwenties. When I wasn't with Libby, I was getting to know Erika, the survivor I'd first seen on the website. She posed for the cover each year. As we'd talk, laugh, and not be afraid to pass gas in front of each other, I began to experience what, I imagined, Molly had found in Amanda. It had been hard feeling like a unicorn all my life. A colon cancer survivor—at my age—didn't exist. Yet in the company of fellow unicorns, I felt both unique and the same. I wasn't the only twentysomething girl with long hair and an even longer vertical scar.

"Danielle, you're up!"

Although we weren't *real* models, like the ones walking runways just a few hours south in New York City, the Colon Club wanted us to feel as though we were. They taped a casting call with our names and photo shoot times to the door of a makeshift hair and makeup room. From having my wardrobe picked out to getting ideas for makeup and hair, it did feel awesome to be pampered. I'd never identified as a model in my life (and found it ironic that I was being treated like one, considering my teenage quest to compare myself to them). I wasn't sure if I'd ever dreamed of *being* a model when I was younger, or just *looking* like one.

It took a few hours of curling my long, dark hair, applying heavy makeup, and styling my clothes to get me ready for the photographer. Technically, his studio was a recently tidied garage with lawn equipment and boxes either pushed to the sides or shelved. Yet Mark McCarty was a total pro, and his skill level was obvious. Whether he was shooting in some of the priciest city spaces or a lake house garage, he had a gift for capturing the essence and spirit of his subjects.

"Stand here. Look this way. Perfect, ohhhh. Wow-www. Gorgeous. Stunning."

His compliments were unending and appreciated. They helped me feel less awkward. I already felt like a million bucks thanks to the pampering, but Mark, his assistant, and the graphic designer, Troy, made me feel like two million. I was no stranger to having my picture taken; I had a mom who documented nearly all my life. Yet this was a little different from the candid shots on the playground or me opening birthday presents. I was standing on a backdrop with big, black umbrella light shades while a solo shooter getting multiple angles kept asking me to give him a variety of poses and faces.

"Okay, lift up your shirt and show us that scar."

I had known the moment was coming before I ever stepped onto the airplane. It was the Way of the Colondar, something each model did. Our long, vertical scars tied us together (especially because laparoscopic surgeries were slowly being adopted by surgeons and not too common yet). Our scars were like armor. Our weapons of warfare against cancer were, first and foremost, our bodies. I knew when I received the invitation to pose in the Colondar that I'd be asked to reveal it.

Our scars were like armor. Our weapons of warfare against cancer were, first and foremost, our bodies.

But I hesitated. It wasn't a no-brainer decision. I'd experienced such an odd relationship with my scar over the years. I didn't know if I wanted it public. Thinking it looked ugly, I wanted to hide the scar with one-piece swimsuits and not talk about it. But over time, as it faded from red to pink to white, I began to appreciate its purpose and its story. It helped save my life. Although I'd become okay with the idea of revealing my scar, I was struggling to show off parts of my body. To thousands. Of strangers.

Beyond the surface-level fears of lifting up my shirt and appearing too white or too pudgy was an even bigger discomfort. "Waist down" had not only become my two most hated words, they caused me to freeze anytime a man I didn't know very well asked to see parts of my otherwise covered body. I'd received more rectal exams in one year than most men got in a lifetime (leaving no room for empathy when it came to them avoiding cancer checks because of "turn and cough" fears). When I was asked to reveal *any* skin, including my abdomen, anxiety ran through my chest, and my stomach started churning.

Yet Mark had said it, I had known it was coming, and instead of quitting, I wanted to push through. I hadn't flown all this way to not show my scar. I replayed in my mind *why* I was doing the calendar—to help people know that young people like me can get colon cancer and to inspire other teen girls struggling with embarrassment to not hide what's happening with their bodies. I took a deep breath to pause, made the decision to be brave, then slowly lifted up the bottom hem of my black tank top and offered a Mona Lisa–type smile to the camera.

May 31, 2008
I'm in NY at the Colondar photo shoot. What a

road it has been to get here. Everyone is unique in that our ages and situations really vary. I'm one of the youngest here, but also one of the furthest into remission. It's been neat to hear so many people's stories and see what they're going through even now. Not only does being here bring back memories from when I was sick, but it's also bringing back memories of my journey to seven years. I'm not sure I would be as active as the others who are here only after a few months or years. I'm inspired.

"Hey, you should apply!"

I checked my Facebook notifications to read a message from David, another Colondar model. What I hadn't realized when I agreed to do the Colondar was that I'd be joining a big "model family." With both models past and models to come, I would experience a sorority effect where no matter what year they modeled for the Colondar, we'd be in the same club. This club had become invaluable a few months after my Colondar released. Cancer Round 2 hit and fellow survivors rallied around me.

I'd kept writing on my blog, and as I made friends with people inside the community, my following grew—as did my opportunities. When Colon Club staff realized I was experienced in public relations and could write well, they asked if I'd help out, and I gladly volunteered. At first, I took on writing press releases. Then, I began returning to Lake George each year so I could meet the models personally and write their bios. I was thrilled to use my PR degree for the very reason I'd obtained it—I wanted to give back to cancer by way of communications.

David and I were connected on Facebook because he too was a Colondar model who lived in the Midwest. He'd noticed a flyer about a photo shoot in Kansas City posted by another nonprofit, Fight Colorectal Cancer— or, as people nicknamed it, Fight CRC. They were looking for survivors to participate.

"Maybe; we'll see," I typed back. It's not that I wasn't up for sharing my story, but between juggling a freelance marketing business I'd begun after transitioning away from church staff, volunteering with the Colon Club, and leading small group, my plate felt full. Not to mention I was balancing being a wife to Mike and had become a mom to a now-Dora the Explorer–loving toddler all at the same time.

Yet something about the opportunity was hard to shake, and as I prayed about it one night, I felt a nudge to go. In the midst of a lot of spinning plates, I didn't want to forget my story. My purpose for still being alive. If my life could help inspire or encourage another, it gave meaning to why I enjoyed survivorship. Life felt fuller when I was keenly aware that each day is truly a gift, and no part of it, including tomorrow, is ever guaranteed.

After falling asleep pondering the photo shoot, I emailed the next morning. "Hi, I'm a colon cancer survivor in Kansas City—was diagnosed at ages seventeen and twenty-five. Let me know if you need more survivors!"

I got a near-instant reply. "Yes, we'd love to have you at our photo shoot!" It was signed Anjee Davis, VP of programs (She would later become Fight CRC's president).

A few weeks later, I found myself stepping into another photo shoot and in front of another backdrop. This time I wasn't in a garage in Lake George but on the third floor of a brick building in downtown Kansas City. Timid. A little nervous. I wanted to clam up and be shy. But then I saw Belle and instantly felt more at ease.

"Isn't this great?" Her big smile beamed. "I love this group. Me and the kids went to DC with them last March and learned how to advocate!"

A fellow Colondar model, I'd met Belle on the wraparound porch overlooking Lake George. Like most everyone else in her life, I adored her. Her enthusiasm and gentle spirit were intoxicating. She was just as sweet as her name. If Belle trusted an organization enough to fly her family from Portland, Oregon, to Kansas City to participate, I could trust them too.

The afternoon flew by, and I briefly connected with other models and members of Fight CRC's staff, making sure to meet Michael, the guy who used Twitter and liked to talk tech. Aware of the time (and needing to pick up Mae from day care at my stepmom's by around five o'clock), I didn't stay long to chitchat once my photos and video were finished. I figured they'd fill me in on where they were going and how they'd be used later.

"Would you be interested in blogging for us?"

I laughed at the request, not because I didn't want to

do it, and not because it was funny, but because I was a little beside myself that the blog I'd started to help me cope with Cancer Round 2 had become an avenue to getting so deeply involved in the cancer community. While my story helped crack open doors for me, my ability to write well blew them wide open. I kept reading the message from Anjee: "We need help when March, Colorectal Cancer Awareness Month, comes . . . we can pay you."

I froze—pay me? For cancer awareness? This was a little new. All the awareness I'd done up to this point with my story had been, gladly, volunteered. The Colon Club depended on grassroots volunteers like me. All the staff and board donated our time and gave our stories away. Yet Fight CRC was a little different. They had a paid staff, sponsors, and a much, much bigger organization. As a freelancer and young mom, I was intrigued by their offer.

I asked for more details, and soon Anjee sent over her ideas. They were about to launch a campaign called One Million Strong on March 1 in Times Square. It would have an inflatable colon (inspired by Molly's original crawl-through idea) that people could walk through, a dance party, yoga, and giveaways. Dozens of volunteers were planning to show up dressed in head-to-toe blue, and they needed someone to pull together pictures and excerpts from the event and write up a recap blog post.

It seemed simple enough, and I was in the habit of blogging a lot. I agreed to write the post, and when the first day of March arrived, I woke up to an early alarm. While Mae slept soundly in her toddler bed, I started flipping back and forth between *Good Morning America* and the *Today Show* and spotted the group's volunteers waving their signs high in the air. I logged on to social media to get an even better idea of the event, amazed that I could follow along with something happening in Times Square. Technology had bridged such a gap, and now what was happening in New York City was directly impacting me in my Kansas City living room.

Major media outlets took notice of the "stunt"—an inflatable colon in Times Square was big news. By midday, I noticed a few headlines covering the event and sifted through the posted photos. It was exciting to have even a small part in what was happening, that is, until I realized my role was actually jumbo-sized.

"Is that you?"

I had a Facebook notification from Anjee; she'd tagged me in a picture. I clicked to load it, and there I was—my photo and video from the shoot on the Nasdaq Jumbotron. A huge picture of *my* face was being broadcast into Times Square.

"What in the WORLD!" Completely speechless, it was *my* photo in one of the most visited, beauty-obsessed spots in the world. Sandwiched between rotating ads featuring America's top models, Coke, and Broadway shows was me—Danielle, the midwestern girl who survived colon cancer at age seventeen! Wow. I didn't think posing for the Colondar and hearing that thousands of people pinned up my Colondar picture to their walls would ever be topped. But here I was four short years later, and the impact of my personal story seemed to only be getting bigger.

"Can you write for Call-On Congress too?"

Not even a week had passed between finishing the blog post for Fight CRC and receiving the request to write another. I appreciated the gesture and assumed it meant Fight CRC liked my work.

"I could . . . but it might be difficult if I'm not there."

I really wanted to do the project, but it had been challenging to encapsulate the details from New York City when I was watching it unfold primarily through social media. I sensed there was more happening at the event, like survivors stopping by and people reacting as they walked through a colon, that could be told only by experiencing it.

"I'll get you to DC."

Disbelief was a theme, and I once again couldn't believe Anjee's response. Was a client really offering to fly me to Washington, DC, to write about an event for a series of blog posts? Yes, yes indeed. I wasn't dreaming. I wanted to give Anjee an instant okay, but pitter-patters of little feet against our hardwood floors reminded me I couldn't just go in and out of town without talking it over with my family, even if it was for work. I was already leaving for a week in the summer to be at the next Colondar shoot. This would require another several days away from home. Mike had to be in agreement with it since it put him on full-time parenting.

When we were dating, I assumed Mike would make a great dad, and when I watched him as a teacher, that solidified it. His calm demeanor and genuine investment in others, as well as his propensity to build a team and his loyalty to stick with it, got me excited to watch him in action. It was heartwarming to actually see him become daddy to Mae. Daddy dates became a top priority, and it wasn't unusual for him to take her on adventures in the park or give her lessons on recognizing and listing to good music. Shortly after we adopted Mae, he left teaching to work for my friend Amy D., a fellow Christian who owned a website company. She was so supportive of our family that he felt like we could make it work.

"You can't not take this opportunity," Mike insisted as we talked over Anjee's offer and the mom guilt I instantly felt for considering it. It was hard enough not staying at home like my own mom when I was young (although running my own business and working from home did make me really available). But we thought our life would slow down once we finalized Mae's adoption. It had felt like life was a revolving door between graduating college, getting married, my parents each getting remarried, lining up jobs, changing jobs, starting a church, starting a business, facing a second cancer, and adopting. We were ready to settle down. Me traveling for work? That wasn't part of our plans. Yet, maybe, they were part of God's?

"God's going to take care of us," Mike often reminded me. I knew he was right. God was in charge of our future, not me. When I saw the decision more as discerning God's plan for my life, not my own, the answer became clear. Only He could have opened *this* door. So a few weeks later, I boarded an airplane bound for Reagan International Airport.

I had an extra gusto in my step thanks to a call from

Dr. Geier. Apparently, the gene that had always been declared a "variant of unknown significance" (a.k.a. "the fluke") had been reclassified by the lab thanks to more patient data, giving me a genetic syndrome. The variant showing up in my tumors was *very* significant. I officially had Lynch syndrome, and I carried a gene mutation putting me at high risk for not only colon, but several other cancers. Fortunately, my doctors suspected this after Cancer Round 2, and they'd treated me like a Lynch patient anyway. But the news didn't only offer an answer to the why questions of my cancers. It awakened me to the somber reality: I'd never be out of the woods with cancer for the rest of my life. I had to grieve and find acceptance.

Coping came relatively easily, though, as I joined nearly a hundred people gathered in our nation's capital for a week dedicated to saving, lengthening, and improving colorectal cancer patient lives. I was there to work and find the stories, yet walking around with a personal history inevitably connected me to the people. I made more new friends, both with the advocates and Fight CRC's staff, and I began to feel like I'd found my destiny.

"This feels like I'm doing what I was made to do," I journaled from my hotel room after the last night.

I made more new friends, both with the advocates and Fight CRC's staff, and I began to feel like I'd found my destiny.

Something inside me had come alive; purpose was beginning to overlay so many years of pain.

"We want to hire you as our director of communications."

I'd hoped Anjee would ask me to do more projects once March settled down, but a full-time job offer with a salary and benefits? It came as a shock, yet it felt like the job was uniquely designed and perfectly created for me.

"You're seriously offering my dream job. This is exactly what I went to college to do," I told Anjee. And while Mike and I had another talk to weigh the pros and cons, similar to the one before I left for DC, we couldn't turn it down—especially with the promise of flexibility, virtual working from Kansas City, and mutual understanding from one working mom to another (Anjee's son was just a year older than Mae).

"But heads-up—March is crazy."

I was up for the challenge.

I took the job and quickly found out Anjee wasn't joking. Planning for the next year began immediately. It was jarring at first. Living under a cancer cloud meant I rarely planned more than a few months out. But to organize national campaigns, we had to look nine to twelve months ahead. Fortunately, I wasn't working alone. We had an incredible team.

"Small but mighty" is what we considered ourselves, and "strong" began to epitomize all we did. The One Million Strong campaign was taking off after its kickoff, the Times Square event left both good impressions and big shoes. We got to work right away, dreaming up how to get the public's attention and fill the world with awareness messages. As it turns out, just weeks after coming on board, singer/songwriter (and fellow Missourian!) Sheryl Crow hooked up with us for a video interview, which became our next year's celebrity PSA and cover story for our newly created magazine, *Beyond Blue*.

Year after year for several that followed, celebrities with a personal connection became willing to use their spotlights and shine a light on our cause, a "taboo" cancer that was often not addressed. I'd answer each email, phone call, and invitation professionally, yet behind the scenes still try to comprehend what exactly was happening. From bomb-sniffing dogs that would need to be present at our NYC Grand Central Terminal event to interviews with *Today Show* producers and attending Stand Up to Cancer in Los Angeles, my life had come a long way from the suburbs of Missouri. As each month went on, I (erroneously) doubted the once-in-a-lifetime moments could be topped.

March 20, 2014

Today, I went to the White House. I loved the floral arrangements on each one of the tables—they are fresh every day and so pretty! They reminded me of my wedding bouquet. We saw President Obama's dog getting walked on the lawn, and I picked up one of Michelle's recipes before we left. The rooms were really white and clean. A lot was roped off that we couldn't see. I can't believe I got to tour it today.

From Times Square to the White House steps, colorectal cancer opened so many unbelievable doors. A news article that was published about my thirtieth birthday was picked up and syndicated around the globe. The PR girl in me especially lit up when outlets like *Newsweek* and the *Washington Post* responded to our press releases, and when reality TV show producers called to collaborate. I'd walked the Daytona Speedway track for a photo shoot with a survivor and talked about young adult colorectal cancer (diagnoses under age fifty) on Nashville's Country Music Hall of Fame stage. The job often felt more like dreaming versus working—at least sometimes. It was fun, but we worked so hard.

Big opportunities kept coming, and I reminded myself: they weren't springing up out of nowhere. As our campaigns skyrocketed, so did our hours. A yearning to save the world drove our small staff that kept growing. I began to hire students from my alma mater's public relations program. Andrew, Elizabeth, and I made up a small but powerful communications team. We nearly lived at our computers for several months leading up to March, blurring the lines between days and nights. After a few years into the job, I had rolled my suitcase down so many airport terminals, I eventually lost count how many. And while all of it felt exciting and I'd be giddy about each new opportunity, I couldn't deny the demands of the job were taking a toll.

My body was struggling to keep up—I faced diarrhea, dehydration, and fatigue nearly every time I flew. Mentally and emotionally, I was wearing down. Meeting a community of fighters built me up so much, yet losing them knocked me down. Triggered by the trauma of loss from cancer, in addition to feeling guilt over being one who survived (why me and not them?), I knew I had to slow down. My body, heart, soul, and mind were begging for it. But I really didn't want to.

I was made for this! I told myself as I'd push to keep going, keep working, and keep advocating. I'd reasoned that if traveling to Jamaica to build houses and starting churches in Kansas City weren't my mission fields, God was using me in the cancer community. This was the mission field, the ministry, I'd looked for all along.

I didn't exactly love its rite of passage—a personal connection—but I couldn't deny God was using me! I was a light getting sent into unbelievable places, a light in total denial about my flickering.

22

Home

"HOW DO YOU DO HER hair?"
I started to travel a lot for work when Mae was age three, yet thanks to the flexibility of Fight CRC and the empathy of several other parents on staff, I was gone for just a few days at a time, and it was a priority to keep me at home as much as possible. When at home, I'd play princess dress up or read books with my girl. When we'd run errands, not only would Mae quickly compliment strangers, but strangers would also come up to her. Usually, I could anticipate their comment. It would have to do with her cuteness or her hair.

From her earliest baby days to when she became a rumbling, tumbling toddler and then an elementary school girl, Mae's iconic hair was a showstopper. A puffy poof of soft, beautiful coiled curls was an instant way to find her in a crowd. Both strangers and close friends alike were enchanted by her. Not only were the gorgeous locks memorable, they intrinsically carried our family's unique story. With her curly hair and mocha skin contrasted against my porcelain, freckled skin and Mike's tan yet very Caucasian complexion, it was obvious that we were different. Most accurately assumed we'd become a family through adoption. I never minded repeating our September story.

Thinking back, when I was younger, I viewed the suburban setting of my hometown as boring. But once Mike and I settled down (and felt called by God to stay), I began to understand why my parents moved. With a growing girl of our own, we began to appreciate what the family-friendly suburbs had to offer. Although it was challenging to be different at times, I hoped our family could help bring awareness and openness to not only adoption, but diversity.

Instead of seeing the thriving blue-ribbon schools, revitalized downtown, and well-kept parks as a bore, I suddenly appreciated these important facets of our community. Our hometown had continued to grow and expand since Mike's and my elementary and high school days, though some things never changed. For example, the downtown diner still served appetizer cinnamon rolls. And in over twenty years, nobody had outdone outlaw Cole Younger; he remained one of our biggest claims to fame. (His grave happened to be just a few miles down from the Corner of Monroe.) I chuckled that Mae, too, would go on to learn about an infamous outlaw at school and wonder how to make her own mark on the world. I was certain about one thing: it was going to be different from mine.

Growing up with a little brother like Andy prepared me for raising a daughter like Mae. She wasn't boisterous and rowdy like him, but she carried her own bold, sassy, creative personality. She was very different from me. Even as a mom, I tended to be quieter, calm, and hid my emotions well. Not my Mae. She wasn't afraid to be loud and be seen. Not as a baby. Not as a second grader yelling "Hello!" to her friends out the car window. She carried a confidence I was still learning how to find. But that wasn't all.

Early on, Mae loved feeling fancy and looking girly as she draped herself in beaded necklaces and wigs. You wouldn't have found a single Barbie doll in my childhood bedroom, but they filled up Mae's toy room and Christmas lists. The backyard park and basketball court presented all sorts of adventures for me, but for Mae, her adventure was a setup in her toy room she named Barbie City.

Mae didn't need books, movies, siblings, or neighbor kids to help her make believe and have fun. All she needed was her imaginative mind. At age two, she began developing characters and turned anything she put her hands on into them. It didn't matter whether they were plastic figurines or simply forks, spoons, and knives. *Every*thing could become a family (most of the time girls only) in her eyes.

Early on, I knew our minds worked differently; her lens in which she viewed the world had a far different bend. Not only was she extremely creative, but she was growing up as a biracial adopted kid raised by two white parents. Yet Mike and I had decided to embrace the differences and stay open about both her race and adoption. Connecting often with her birth mom's family and individuals in the African American community, we wanted to celebrate that we didn't look alike and not ignore it.

"She's going to grow up in a world seeing and experiencing things differently from you," Barbara continually reminded me out of both her experience as a licensed therapist *and* as a woman of color. She helped plant seeds of confidence that I could do it. I had what it took. I could be a good mom to Mae. I had so much to learn, but I made sure to do one thing: embrace hard conversations.

They sprang up in kindergarten around Martin Luther King Jr. Day, when Mae got her first history lesson on his famous "I Have a Dream" speech and the sad story about colored and white water fountains. Inspired by Dr. King, she and her classmates had been encouraged to write their own dreams.

> I have a dream that bullying will stop. I will stop it by standing up for people that are being bullied and be kind.
> *—MAE*

I couldn't have been prouder. Not long after, the questions came.

"If it was the olden days, could I have drunk out of the white water fountains?"

"If we were born a long time ago, would people have wanted you to adopt me?" The thought of raising a little girl brought the assumption that, like my life, discussing puberty would be one of the hardest mother-daughter talks we'd face. But I thought wrong. Discussing the history of race in America proved to be even harder.

"You can tell me anything," I'd constantly remind Mae, feeling thankful when she took me up on it. As we'd discuss tough topics, however, I noticed that both Barbara and Mae seemed to possess something I lacked. They could take in what went wrong, yet quickly forgive and offer limitless grace.

"I've been in church my whole life, and I've never seen a transformation like this."

I sat down in a worn upholstered chair with a used, stained coffee cup in my hand. Stunned and trying to process what I'd just witnessed, I certainly hadn't expected this.

It was my first time attending an AA meeting. I'd only seen and heard about them on TV. Within a few minutes after the meeting began, I realized Hollywood had it both wrong and right. Most people did introduce and label themselves an alcoholic when they got up to the podium.

"Hi. I'm James, and I'm an alcoholic."

"Hi, James."

But what the entertainment industry had failed to show were the incredible stories.

I'd not attended the AA meeting as an alcoholic. I'd been invited by a family member celebrating five years of sobriety who asked the family to come listen to a speech. Having gladly accepted the invitation (I'd prayed for and witnessed the transformation myself!), I'd eagerly taken a seat and begun learning about the Twelve Steps of recovery. I loved hearing the stories about how men and women used them to go from hopeless alcoholic to empowered and free. I'd entered the meeting expecting to encourage others on their journey to sobriety that night, yet I didn't expect to walk out of the meeting so personally moved and inspired to change.

"I can't believe it. Now, that's what it's all about."

Mike was graciously patient, listening to me process what we'd both just heard. I couldn't stop talking.

Sober alcoholics described the trauma they'd faced, why they'd turned to drinking, and the how the Twelve Steps had gotten them out of it. Along the way, they seemed to have found something I was still looking for (when I wasn't working sixty hours a week). The morning after the AA meeting, I began a quest to find it.

Calling Barbara to set up more sessions was easy and relieving. I was grateful for a person to help me find what I seemed to be lacking (a sponsor, as AA would call it). I wasn't quite in the same shape I'd been in when I first sat on her couch and made hand gestures to describe an invisible trauma cake. But some layers of the cake either seemed to still be there or had returned, thanks to what I'd soon learn to call "triggers."

Parenting, no doubt, had triggered some issues, unresolved hurts hiding in my heart. Mae was practically a little mirror walking around, reflecting things I both did and said when I was happy—and angry. I'd undergone a hysterectomy when Mae was eighteen months old, and having my female organs removed (as a preventive surgery) sparked both fears of cancer's return as well as grief. Although I wasn't sad to not get periods anymore, I grieved that I would never, ever, ever produce a human life now (and I couldn't change my mind and call a reproductive specialist). The finality was hard, and once again, I needed to learn to love my body.

And then there was Mike. He had always been, and never stopped being, wonderful. But I had noticed—and eventually he did too—that we'd pulled away from each other after Cancer Round 2. Unaware of it at the time, facing cancer as a twentysomething married couple differed from facing it as teens. Cancer Round 1 drew us together—closer—through love letters, gentle kisses on my forehead, and spur-of-the-moment surprise visits. But Cancer Round 2? It scared the poop out of both of us. Instead of hugs every morning and every night, or a commitment to do everything together (as much as possible), it became easier to go our separate ways. Unattach. We were still together a lot but were not always, or even often, emotionally on the same page. Fortunately, our commitment to believe "God's going to take care of us" (and advice from a few marriage conferences) opened our eyes to what was happening. Appointments with Barbara helped me address what was going on between us and take some steps to mend it.

It was good to routinely see Barbara again, yet also a little strange and confusing. I thought I'd already been through inner healing. Was there more? I didn't really understand. Yet after an hour at the AA meeting, I had a better picture of the true state of my soul. I wasn't where I'd started out when I first called her. I had a good grasp on my faith, but now I needed to learn to apply it. The sober eyes and stories looked so appealing because I'd not yet found what they had. I wanted to; I longed for it. Where to start? Forgive.

I thought I *had* forgiven already, but come to find out, there was more to do. As we dove into even deeper layers of my trauma cake, I had to forgive each piece of the story. My body for making cancer *and* being infertile, the doctors for touching me, my own ego for worshiping a warped body image influenced by magazines, my friends for abandoning me, Mom and Dad for divorcing, Mike for withdrawing. Hardly anyone, including my own self, was immune. But then it happened again. I saw what I needed to address most of all: God. He'd allowed me to suffer so much loss and pain.

Dang it.

It didn't seem right. *Me* forgive *God?* Yet my heart needed to work through the process if I wanted to be close to Him. Little did I realize I'd kept accusing Him of being absent. Neglectful. And because of that, He didn't yet have access to every nook and cranny. Promptly, I forgave Him (and then asked for *His* forgiveness, since my thinking was so warped). It's hard to explain, like the moment I felt God pick me up from the chair at Camp Shamineau, but in a second, I understood God as a Father who sees me as a beloved daughter. I'd found what the sober eyes carried. I felt wholly, totally free.

It's time to move on from Fight CRC.

It's time to move on from Fight CRC.

I quickly came to realize freedom does come with a price. For a while, as a mom, wife, and communications pro, I'd sensed the need to step down from my full-time job growing more urgent. And while the resignation chat with Anjee was hard and sad, everyone understood. She especially got it not only as a working mom herself, but as a close friend. The staff knew one major reason was driving my decision: *home.*

Home. It had been a painful word as a teen. But as God healed both my body and my heart, the word grew on me. The Corner of Monroe was getting harder to leave. Our life was still full of church small groups (reconnecting with Adam from high school led to us joining his church family and making even more Christian friends). For years, we'd offered for friends to live with us, and after a basement remodel, it actually happened. Our friend Nicole, whom we nicknamed Doc, moved in, and we began a journey of community living. Thanks to her expertise from growing up on a farm, we tilled and sowed seeds in a backyard garden, and she brought new varieties of flowers to the yard. A great cook, she also brought new flavors (and vegetable varieties) into our evening dinners, along with many other beautiful things.

To destress, I got hooked on baking. A lesson on homemade pie crust by my mother-in-law gave me confidence that soon flowed into chocolate chip cookies once I found a *perfect* recipe. Biscuits. Brownies. Baked goods galore. It became my way to unwind, a year-round activity I enjoyed. I especially loved it when Mom and I established an annual Christmas baking tradition when

Mae was a toddler. The joy of forming a new holiday routine helped me overlook the mountain of colorful sprinkles atop each sugar cookie cutout.

Home—it had a nice ring to it.

Exciting things were happening at the Corner of Monroe—and beyond. As the idea of home began to take root, it flooded into other relationships. Enough time had passed to heal the wounds of divorce; forgiveness had brought freedom. I actually loved being in a blended family. Mom and Dad were both happy and in love. I appreciated the pact my four parents made when we adopted Mae: nobody wanted to miss out, so they promised no fighting.

As they kept their promise, new traditions and relationships with my stepparents and stepsiblings formed, in addition to fun times with my in-laws. My role as Aunt B continued to grow as a plethora of nieces and nephews joined our family. Mentoring tween and teen girls became a passion, especially with Ashlyn, a mentee I began taking to dinner at age ten. We had recently celebrated her sweet sixteen. Home is where, at the risk of sounding corny, I wanted to be—for a lot of reasons.

> Home is where, at the risk of sounding corny, I wanted to be—for a lot of reasons.

I mean, it was still my preferred place to poop. But at the tip-top of my long list of reasons I wanted to be home was one little mayor of Barbie City, who was getting bigger before my eyes.

I'd blinked, dang it, and found out that people were

years old in just a matter of seconds, or so it seemed. And while I'd been enjoying each step of her getting older, I knew what would soon be on the way. Fourth grade. Girl talks. Body changes. Boys. I wanted nothing more than to help her get through her tween and teen years, and I was willing to give up anything. My job and salary. My time and attention. My privacy.

I was hopeful this little one would not feel shame about puberty or the need to hide her body. To help her, I wanted to tell her my full story. I would lay everything on the table and write it in full, no detail left behind. Should other people read it and be inspired too, well, that was a bonus blessing.

> 5-15-18
> B,
> Thank you for the last five years at Fight CRC. We were so excited then, I never imagined today and that I'd be more excited. I freakin' love you! Thank you for all your hard work. Now share your story! You can do it!
> —Mikey

23

Full Circle

I T WAS A BEAUTIFUL FALL evening, an hour before sundown. The sky broadcast pink and red. Acorns were knock-dropping onto our roof as the oak tree's branches swayed in the wind. I kept mistaking them for hail, though it wasn't raining. Brave baby squirrels kept crawling onto our front porch to snatch up the fresh ones, then quickly scattered back into the bushes as our front glass door swung open and Mae stomped down the front stairs.

"Come on, Molly!" she shouted with such volume that our neighbors two streets down could overhear. Mom's voice from the park had nothing on Mae's.

She had been practicing riding her bike without training wheels, and she was finally ready to show her best friend she could do it. They were both ready to ride. Molly strapped on her unicorn helmet over her long, wavy blond hair. She giggled at the thought of riding of riding down the street with Mae, anticipating a wise crack or two. Mae liked to make her laugh. But Mae was also focused on her helmet, a pink one Daddy had found her that worked with her hair. (Just a few weeks prior, she'd decided that instead of wearing her natural coily hair, she wanted to try long braided extensions. Fortunately, the helmet snugged over the braids.)

The girls walked their bikes to the edge of the street, looked both ways for cars, then hopped on. They reminded me so much of Emily and me more than twenty years prior. Their bikes were even identical. As the girls started pedaling, I sat in the white rocking chair on our porch to keep an eye on them.

"Don't go past Ray's. I can't see your helmets past that house."

I was highly aware I sounded just like my mom when she'd set boundaries for Andy and me in the park, yet it was something I'd come to terms with. If I wanted Mae to find her voice, I had to use mine—which meant that sometimes I would probably sound like my own mother. Yet as I got older, I didn't mind it so much. I was starting to understand, more and more, her point of view. Believe it or not, I didn't think twice about buying toilet paper for the house. Perhaps it was even a sign I was on the right track. Looking back, I could see how I looked up to Mom to be my standard when I was Mae's age—and I hoped my daughter felt the same way about me.

From the porch I looked for flashes of helmets to show me the girls were still safe. They were growing up in a world much different from Andy's and mine, a world where I now, unfortunately, didn't feel comfortable with them riding alone without a parent nearby. A world that no longer could wait until fourth grade to teach girls about puberty and protecting their bodies.

I'd been told by moms of older girls to bump up "the talk" by a few years from when I first heard it, but I hadn't expected to start in on it (in a very age-appropriate way) in kindergarten. Yet the girls were growing up in a culture even more obsessed with beauty and riches than the one in which my cousin Kristi and I came of age, and Mae was coming home from school with questions about terms she'd overheard. Although I loved social media because it kept me in touch with so many friends, like Sarah from the neighborhood and Erin from high school, it also presented a challenge. Either it was going to be me or the internet offering her honest answers. I chose me. Once Mae's first questions began and her interest in growing bodies and girl stuff grew, I tried to anticipate what came next and start the discussions. If there was anything I wanted to pass on to her, it was a plea to not be embarrassed about, hide, or harm her body.

"If you see *anything* weird . . . come tell me. If you see any bleeding when you go poop, I need to be the first to know."

Poop. Butts. Farts. It was all on the table at our house, and as a little girl growing up, she loved it. I tried to train her when *not* to say the words at school, but I was proud. Talking about everything from poop to periods to purity was possible for her at home. My, had I come a long way.

Beeeeeeeep.

The kitchen stove timer went off and I ducked inside for a minute. The house smelled amazing, filling me with pride. Hot vegetable soup simmered on the stove, and the timer was telling me the homemade flakey biscuits were browned. As I opened the oven to snatch out the biscuits—just in time—they were perfectly golden. I let them cool down while I returned to the porch.

"Girls, we're going to eat in a few minutes!"

"Okay, okay!" they yelled back.

It was an uneventful evening at home, and Molly was planning to eat with us. We enjoyed having her, and lots of guests, around our table often. Mike's and my long-held dreams for the Corner of Monroe to be a welcoming place and an open table seemed to be coming true.

I went inside to check the biscuits and turned down the temperature on the soup so we could soon eat. Returning to the porch to check for helmets and give a final "Dinner's ready" warning, I had another idea.

With some wild-wide smiles, Mae and Molly were indeed riding down the street unbound. No more training wheels for these girls. They were tasting pure freedom, the kind that came as a young girl when you started to break away. I didn't want to ruin the moment, I remembered the feeling well, but as a mom I couldn't help myself: "Mae, can I get you on video?"

I knew our friends and family would also want to celebrate the milestone. Despite its vices, social media was good for sharing. I wasn't posting pictures from Times Square or the White House steps anymore, but I'd learned something along the way. Most people were just as excited to celebrate the small victories as they were the big ones. Maybe I didn't work in the same national spotlight as I once had, but cancer survivors, blog readers, friends, and family members kept encouraging me.

"Keep writing! I love your blog!"

The encouragement to keep writing and sharing opened my eyes to my real mission field—not one particular job or church, not even a country. Simply being alive and carrying God's love into every place, to every person—that was what I'd been called to do all along. It was like a light bulb moment—I got it.

"I'm going to do a Facebook Live video, okay? One, two, three, go!"

With one foot on the pedal and the other pushing off from the street just like I'd taught her, Mae hopped onto her bike, and within seconds she and Molly zoomed past me. During the live-streamed video, I commented that whoever paralleled riding a bike with something coming easily obviously hadn't taught many strong-willed nine-year-old girls to ride. It hadn't been an easy process. It had taken weeks of teaching her and then watching her stand up, fall, and try again. But finally, over time, she got it. I couldn't have been prouder.

Once I ended the video, I corralled everyone to the table for dinner. The biscuits were perfect—not too hot yet still warm. While I was scooping soup into colorful bowls, Mae and Molly chose their seats. I loved the slower pace I was learning to live. I'd taken on some freelance projects but worked far fewer hours. It gave me time to bake biscuits and cook dinner on a weeknight, plus freedom to spend fall evenings with my kiddo on our porch. And to write. Not all our evenings were like this one. Sometimes we did have places to go, but when we didn't, I savored it. I wanted more of the slow.

The girls waited for Mike, Doc, and me to dish up our food so we could pray. Yummm. It was good, and well worth the extra time to cook it homemade. What had taken me a few hours to prepare was gone within twenty minutes, but I'd come to expect that. I wasn't sure if I'd always have the patience, or the time, to make dinners like this. But in this season, I was learning to appreciate the process.

Mike and Doc offered to clear the table and clean the kitchen, and the girls ran upstairs to the toy room to play. I took advantage of a brief moment to rest, alone, and stepped back onto the porch.

The breeze was getting cooler, and the sun was going down. Seeing the maroon mums Doc and I had picked out and orange pumpkins on my porch was instantly calming. Something about fall always made me feel sentimental. I'd fallen in love with Mike during the fall, and while I'd experienced other autumn milestones in my life, holding hands with him as we exchanged our first "I love yous" was definitely my favorite. I was grateful to be alive and still with the man who'd insisted I'd see a doctor so long ago, and who had literally saved my behind. This was our story, not just mine.

The squirrels were chasing each other around the yard with just as much energy as the tween girls inside. I marveled at their ability to scale a trunk with effortless intensity as I gazed into the trees. They reminded me of the backyard park behind the yellow house that I'd grown up in. Then and now, trees had always seemed to protect me, looking down to watch me grow.

Did trees like fall? I wondered. Did they appreciate going barren when changing over each year, or even remaining rooted, rock-solid stationary? I didn't really know.

I did know that after they were stripped bare and survived the winter, new life, spring growth, was promised. I knew that for the trees to stay healthy, to house birds, feed squirrels, and offer shade, they had to endure each and every season.

Narrowing my focus on the leaves, I caught sight of it. A distinctive soft pink hue in the fading light. Ha. There was no question. The trees were doing more than tossing a wave down to me on the porch below or bravely, boldly standing tall. They were totally blushing.

ACKNOWLEDGMENTS

MIKEY B, THANK YOU FOR your courage, vulnerability, and permission to share our story as it falls into many hands and will sit on shelves for years to come. You set a high bar for other husbands, but that's a good thing. You're a man of God. I'm so glad you're mine. You were right: God is going to take care of us.

Mae, you are beautiful, loved, and created by God for such a time as this. I can't wait for you to tell your stories. You're my greatest gift.

Mom, thank you for championing and being a key to this story, our story. I'm blessed to be your daughter.

Dad, even in my late thirties, I'm an unapologetic daddy's girl. Thank you for your unfailing love and your kind and gentle heart.

Andy, although we joke around, I can't imagine life without you. You're my longest friend, and I respect you very much. Thank you for always supporting me in everything I've set out to do.

Curt Pesmen, I'll forever remember our conversation that followed our search for Disney's childhood home—it helped me take the idea of writing a book seriously. Thank you for your strong coaching and smart editing. Although I never took the suggestion since I'm not too familiar with Bowie, for the record, readers should know you did suggest chapter 2 be called "Ch-Ch-Changes."

Will Bryan, thank you once again for letting your creativity flow through the canvas of my book cover. I am still in awe of your work. As a thank-you, I promise to bake you more cookies.

Thank you to all of my first-, second-, and third-round editors: Mike, Amy, Doc, Crystal, Ashlyn, Katie, Anjee, Mom, John, Dad, Andy, and Mom and Dad B. Your suggestions made this book better (and accurate, whew!).

Redemption Press, you've helped my dream come true. Thank you for being author advocates and helping *Blush* come to life! Melissa Hanberry, thank you for introducing them to me. I pray this book also carries Maggie's legacy.

There are so many people to thank who played a role in this story. I wish I had space to mention and name every single one of you! To all of my grandparents, aunts, uncles, stepsiblings, cousins, second cousins, in-laws, nieces, nephews, neighbors, hospital visitors, coworkers, clients, medical teams, colleagues, teachers, fellow Colon Club models, Fight CRC advocates, HACWN writers, high school friends, college friends, church friends, my parents' friends, and more—thank you!

Avenue family, you hold a special place in my heart and this story. It would not have been written without you, and I cherish each one of you dearly.

Navah family, you've offered grace, uttered so many prayers for this project, and helped me find confidence in my voice—not to mention the prophetic pieces of my story. Thank you for helping me find home and beauty. Bless you, my friends!

Jesus, thank You for saving my life and calling me to be a communicator for Christ. Like the woman at the well, my deepest hope is for my story to lead others to encounter You for themselves and believe.